NAET: SAY GOOD-BYE TO ASTHMA

By

Devi S. Nambudripad,

M.D., D.C., L.Ac., Ph.D. (Acu.)

Author of

Say Good-Bye to ... series

THIS BOOK WILL REVOLUTIONIZE
THE PRACTICE OF ASTHMA TREATMENT

The doctor of the future will give no medicine,
But will interest his patients
In the care of the human frame, in diet,
And in the cause and prevention of disease
-Thomas A. Edison

Published by
Delta Publishing Company
6714 Beach Blvd.
Buena Park, CA 90621
(888) 890-0670, (714) 523-8900, Fax: (714) 523-3068
Web site: www.naet.com

DEDICATION

This book is dedicated to patients suffering from Asthma, Allergies and other Lung disorders.

First Edition, 2003

Library of Congress Control No: 2003114400

ISBN: 0-9743915-1-4

Printed in U.S.A.

The medical information and procedures contained in this book are not intended as a substitute for consulting your physician. Any attempt to diagnose and treat an illness using the information in this book should come under the direction of an NAET physician who is familiar with this technique. Because there is always some risk involved in any medical treatment or procedure, the publisher and author are not responsible for any adverse effects or consequences resulting from the use of any of the suggestions or procedures in this book. Please do not use this book if you are unwilling to assume the risks. All matters regarding your health should be supervised by a qualified medical professional.

Contents

Acknowledgement

I am deeply grateful to my husband, Dr. Kris Nambudripad, for his encouragement and assistance in my schooling and, later, in the formulation of this project. Without his cooperation in researching reference work, revision of manuscripts, word processing and proofreading, it is doubtful whether this book would have ever been completed.

My sincere thanks also go to the many clients who have entrusted their care to me, for without them I would have had no case studies, no feedback, and certainly no extensive source of personal research upon which to base this book.

I am also deeply grateful to Meg Brazil, Shirley Reason, Joyce Baisden, Michael Magrutsch, Jean E., Joan E., Torry E., Nita P., Gene F., Marina L., George W., George M., Ron M., Barbara M., Dolores C., Debbie H., Bill H., Toni C., Lucia C., Fiz M., to name a few among many of my devoted asthmatic patients, for believing in me from the very beginning of the research until the present, and by supporting my theory and helping me to conduct the ongoing detective work.

I also have to express my thanks to my son, Roy, who assisted me in many ways in the writing of this book.

Additionally, I wish to thank Robert Prince, M.D., Doretta Zemp, Chi Yu, Fong Tien and many of my associates, who wish to remain anonymous for proofreading and assisting me with this work, and Mr. Sri at Delta Publishing for his printing expertise. I am deeply grateful for my professional training and the knowledge and skills acquired in classes and seminars on chiropractic and kinesiology at the Los Angeles College of Chiropractic in Whittier which is called now the Southern University of Health Sciences, California; the California Acupuncture College in Los Angeles; SAMRA University of Oriental Medicine, Los Angeles; University of Health Sciences, School of Medicine, Antigua; and the clinical experience obtained at the clinics attached to these colleges.

My special thanks also go to Mala Moosad, N.D., R.N., L.Ac., Ph.D., Mohan Moosad, M.S., N.D., D.Ac, who supported and stood by me from the very beginning of my NAET discovery and ongoing research. They helped immensely by taking over my work load at the clinic so that I could complete the book. I also would like to acknowledge my thanks to my dear mother for forever nourishing me emotionally and nutritionally. My heartfelt thanks also go to Dr. Marilyn Chernoff, Barbara Cesmat, Sister Nina, and Margaret Wu, NAET trained practitioners, who have dedicated their time to help desperate allergy sufferers by assisting me in many ways to promote my mission of making NAET available to every needy person not only in this country, but in third world countries as well. I would also like to acknowledge my everlasting thanks to my office manager, Janna Gossen, who worked with me from the first day of my practice of two decades and to Sarah Cardinas, Art Martinez and Athira Suresh and all other staff members for their support.

I would like to remember the late Dr. Richard F. Farquhar at Farquhar Chiropractic Clinic in Bellflower, California. I was a student of chiropractic and acupuncture when I was doing preceptorship with him. When I told him about my NAET discovery, he tried the treatment on himself and was amazed with the results. Then he encouraged me to practice NAET with needles on all his patients. Because of his generosity, I had the opportunity to treat hundreds of patients soon after I discovered NAET.

I do not have enough words to express my heartfelt thanks and appreciation to the California Acupuncture State Board for supporting NAET from the beginning, permitting me to teach other licensed acupuncturists by instantly making me a CEU provider.

Perhaps the California Acupuncture State Board will never know how much they have helped humanity by validating my new technique and allowing me to share the treatment method with other practitioners and, through them, to the countless number of patients like me, who now live normal lives. I am forever indebted to acupuncture and Oriental medicine. Without this knowledge, I myself, would still be living in pain. Thank you for allowing me to share my experience with the world!

I do not have enough words to express my admiration and gratitude to Dr. Sue Gavallas, the director of post graduate department, and Dr. Karen Numeroff, at the College of Chiropractic, Life University, Marietta, Georgia, for making it possible for me to teach NAET to other chiropractors through their college.

I extend my sincere thanks to these great teachers and mentors. They have helped me to grow immensely at all levels. My mentors are also indirectly responsible for the improvement of my personal health as well as that of my family, patients, and the health of other NAET practitioners and their countless patients.

Many of my professors, doctors of Western and Oriental medicine, allopathy, chiropractic, kinesiology, as well as nutritionists, were willing to give of themselves by teaching and committing personal time, through interviews, to help me complete this book. I will always be eternally grateful to them. They demonstrated the highest ideals of the medical profession.

Devi S. Nambudripad, M.D., D.C., L.Ac., Ph.D.(Acu.)

Foreword

Paul Honan, M.D.
Lebanon, Indiana

As occurs with many asthmatics, I outgrew my childhood asthma. It returned as severe 24-hour year-round asthma in 1987. For ten years I struggled with the best of what conventional medicine had to offer and found it wanting. As a physician, I thought I could find access to the best in medicine. Only minor relief of symptoms and avoidance of foods and inhalants to which I was allergic was offered as a treatment. Even so, I had several attacks of anaphylaxis (an anaphylaxis is a life-threatening allergic reaction, characterized by an immediate allergic reaction that can cause difficulty in breathing or severe asthma, lightheadedness, fainting, sensation of chills, internal cold, irregular heart beat, pallor, eyes rolling, poor mental clarity, tremors, internal shaking, extreme fear, throat swelling, drop in blood pressure, redness and hives, fever, delirium, unresponsiveness, etc.)

In 1997, I met ophthalmologist Peter Holyk, M.D. who introduced me to Nambudripad Allergy Elimination Techniques (NAET). After he treated me with basic four NAET treatments, he treated me for sugar. That treatment was remarkable. My asthma improved. Then I attended Dr. Nambudripad's NAET training course and eliminated about 40 other allergies. Since then I have had no more attacks of anaphylaxis.

Over the years, I have joked with Dr. Devi Nambudripad saying that she ruined my comfortable professional life. I had been satisfied thinking I was practicing state-of-the-art medicine. But when she introduced NAET and the wonderful world of energy medicine, my professional practice would never be the same.

My major personal interest has been in the treatment of asthma with NAET. NAET is utilized in many wonderful ways in my medical practice. Using NAET, I have now helped hundreds of asthma sufferers to lead better lives.

Dr. Devi is my hero!

Paul Honan, M.D.
1720 North Lebanon Street,
Lebanon, Indiana

Preface

My realization that NAET could reverse symptoms and triumph over asthma occurred in 1985, years before I could put M.D. after my name. I had recently received my chiropractic license. Ravi and Sina, two friends from my hometown of Chelakkara, India, had come to visit me in California. During their overnight stay, Ravi almost died from an asthmatic attack. The rest, as we say here in America, is history. By 1985, I had been practicing NAET on myself and my family for over a year and was thrilled with the results. In fact, I was still in a daze about the whole thing.

The "rest," is by now thousands of previous asthma sufferers whose symptoms have been greatly diminished or completely reversed by NAET. Today NAET, as practiced by more than 7,500 health practitioners in the United States and around the world, has saved countless lives and kept them free of symptoms. These people have been transformed from being patients who experienced episodes of wheezing, breathlessness, tightness of chest, and suffocating throat constrictions back to living normal lives.

Asthma is the ninth leading cause of hospitalization nationally. Over one billion dollars is spent each year on health care for asthma. By traditional methods, many patients must take medication every day to control symptoms and prevent attacks.

NAET doesn't rely on traditional methods and medication. Instead, NAET utilizes the insights of many disciplines including chiropractic, Oriental medicine, Western physiology and physics, immunology, environmental medicine, and genetics. In its most simplistic terms, NAET reverses energy blockages in the body. When energy is freely flowing along the energy pathways, illness is kept at bay. Blockages occur because a person's immune system responds to normally harmless substances as if they were a threat to the body. To combat these substances, the body forms antigen-antibody complexes. When trying to destroy these complexes, the immune system brings about an autoimmune reaction that can inflame and destroy healthy tissue, which can result in numerous ailments, including asthma.

Since childhood, I was made to understand that I had to be on medication for the rest of my life for constant, nagging pain, body and joint aches. I didn't expect anything else to change my prognosis. Yes, I had experienced the magical results from aspirin and other analgesics, but nothing had been permanent. On certain days, I had to take aspirin every two hours just to keep going. Otherwise, I would have to spend the day in bed, unable to move.

After suffering from myriad illnesses throughout my life, taking Western and Eastern medicine without a break from infancy, a simple acupuncture procedure – a "gift" – offered insight into how I could be free from my chronic illnesses. This was something hard to comprehend for a mind that, by then, had been trained purely in Western medicine. It was this procedure that began my search into helping others become free of the ailments and pain they suffer.

This "gift" came in 1983 while I was an acupuncture student: I had reacted violently to eating a few pieces of raw carrot. I used acupuncture needles on myself to hopefully overcome the severe reactions. Then I laid in bed for 45 minutes. Some of the pieces of carrots were, unknown to me, sticking to my body. When the needle session was complete, I surprisingly found that I no longer reacted to carrot. In fact, as I later discovered, that treatment – acupuncture while in contact with an allergen – took care of my reaction to carrots permanently.

I could not explain how this worked. I asked my acupuncture professors and they didn't have any answers either. Something like this had never happened. One of the professors called my result, "Power of the mind." In his view, it would only work for people who have good control of their minds and, according to him, I was one of those people. Somehow I knew this was not the case. Over the next months I then used this treatment on both my husband and son, both of whom had been experiencing severe reactions to other substances – and it worked! This prompted me to search the libraries and "pick the brains" of the experts to find more about brain anatomy, physiology and biochemistry. (There were no Internet connections to make my search easier.)

I began treating patients in my new acupuncture/chiropractic practice with what I then called NAET (Nambudripad's Allergy Elimination Treatment). Everyone got free treatments because I was still experimenting with the procedure. I didn't feel right to charge them for experimental treatments. In just a few months, I became very busy. I was seeing patients with many different health problems all day, every day. Most of my patients had been pure allopathic (Western medicine) patients who were not satisfied with the results they were getting from their medical doctors. They all wanted "that special experimental treatment."

Soon, referral patients came not only from the United States, but from various parts of India, Europe, Russia, Singapore, Canada, and Israel. Whoever said word of mouth patient referrals are the best was right. My practice has proven that.

I was a willing worker and explorer. I accepted whoever came to my office with whatever health problem. I tested each one for any possible allergic involvement in their condition. Initially, I spent hours on certain people testing all the samples I could get, looking for clues about the causes of the problems they were having. I was becoming convinced on one thing by then – that some kind of allergy was the cause of so many of the human illnesses we see around us. And as I kept looking for allergies in my patients, I found them, treated them right away, and the results convinced me I was right in my assumption that so many human illnesses start with some form of allergy.

I found that almost everyone who came to me suffered from a long list of food allergies. Amazingly, after receiving NAET treatments for their common everyday foods (bread, rice, vegetables, milk, meat, salt, spices, chocolate, etc.) they all noticed huge differences in their health. They reported: *Backache of 30 years is gone... migraines of 22 years are no more... constant neck and shoulder pains are gone... headaches that started after a whiplash 12 years ago is completely relieved... after treatment for tomato, I recovered from cerebral palsy... indigestion is completely relieved.* A patient who was diagnosed with multiple sclerosis at one of the nearby university hospitals went into remission from MS soon after she completed the NAET treatment for basics and nuts, and after 19 years is still in remission. An Italian patient had suffered from angina several times a day for years in spite of taking nitroglycerine regularly. I found him allergic to wine and cheese, which were affecting his heart meridian. I suggested that he avoid wine and cheese for a few days. (Can you imagine what happens when you advise an Italian to give up his wine and cheese?) With great difficulty, he did for the 25 hours it takes for NAET to clear energy pathways (meridians), after which he reported that his angina pains were gone. When Helen, a 79-year-old patient reported to me with tears of joy in her eyes that her *40 years of pancreatitis was no more* I didn't have words to express my gratitude to God for granting me NAET.

Even now not a day passes without saying Wow! At least once when I see the amazing results in my patients. My patients were the true teachers of NAET. I have come a long way from 20 years ago when I began the experimental treatments. At that time, I had nowhere to look for answers, no books to read on this subject, I couldn't discuss it with any professionals nor even my colleagues because no one had heard of anything like this before. No one thought anything like this would be possible – to get completely free from any allergy or allergy-related health disorder. In the early days, whomever I talked to simply shook their heads and said, "Impossible."

Before 1985, I hadn't treated any asthma patients because no one had come to me with that complaint. Then one evening in 1985 after I had just returned from a long day's work, my husband Kris and I got a call from the airport from Ravi and Sina asking if they could visit with us that night since they missed their connecting flight and the next one wasn't available until the following morning. We were happy to bring them from the airport. We hadn't seen them for a few years. So after dinner, we talked until midnight, then reluctantly decided it was time to go to sleep since they had to leave for the airport by seven in the morning.

I was very tired, I fell asleep as soon as I lay down on the bed, but some strange noises woke me up. Some hush-hush talks and heavy breathing coming from the guest room! My husband was still asleep next to me not aware of any noises at all. I waited a few more minutes. I didn't want to intrude upon our guests. But the noises didn't stop. So I came out and saw Sina running between the kitchen and the guest bedroom. She didn't see me approaching since her back was facing my bedroom. She hadn't turned on the lights for fear of waking us up. I looked at the clock. It was only 3:10 a.m., not time for them to leave for the airport.

I walked up to her and asked: Is there any problem Sina?

She startled for a second and said apologetically: "I am sorry, I didn't mean to wake you up. Ravi is having shortness of breath and I didn't know how to help him. I gave him some hot water to drink hoping that will help him. I am scared. He looks horrible."

I turned on the light. At least we could see what was happening under the light now. That woke up my husband too. I like people around me always, then I am not scared.

I looked at Ravi. He was sitting on the bed propped up with pillows at the back. His eyes looked sunken, glassy, and scared. He looked pale and dusky showing that he wasn't getting adequate supply of oxygen. Beads of sweat streamed down his forehead and face. He was perspiring profusely. His undershirt was drenching wet. His breathing was heavy, loud and produced high pitched whistling sound. His airway seemed constricted not letting any air in at all. His radial pulse was very fast and thin, barely palpable. His systolic blood pressure could have been 40 or below, although I didn't waste time to check his blood pressure. Kris (my husband) watched him for a few seconds and said gently "Let's call 911." Kris never gets panicky with anything. He does everything with a relaxed attitude. He walked towards the kitchen counter to reach for the phone.

"Doesn't he carry asthma medication?" I asked his wife.

"He never had asthma before," Sina said. "This is the first time he had this problem."

Ravi wanted to say something but was unable to speak.

But Sina's answer gave me the clue to his present problem.

"Did he eat anything new today that he hasn't eaten before?"

While she was thinking for the answer I was secretly testing using my fingers (Read Chapter 6) to find the culprit of his asthma. I found it. It was in the vitamin C group. More specifically, a fruit... a melon. I asked Ravi," Did you eat any melon today?"

His wife said immediately, "Yes, in the plane we had watermelon. We had never eaten watermelon before. That was the first time he ate that fruit."

In India, watermelon is not a commonly found fruit in some states, especially in my hometown. I had never seen watermelon myself before I came to Los Angeles. I never liked watermelon anyway. I never had an affinity towards that fruit.

I looked at the huge watermelon sitting on the kitchen counter; a patient had earlier brought it as a gift from his garden. (Since I refused to accept payments for my NAET services, some patients insisted on bringing fruits, vegetables, nuts, etc. as gifts.) Then I also remembered that Ravi was sitting a few inches away from the watermelon the whole evening while we were talking. Or shall we say that he was sitting in the electromagnetic field of watermelon while we were conversing for three hours, and the fruit continuously alerting his immune system and the immune system cautioning and calling upon the defense forces to help throw out the dangerous intruder — the watermelon out of his electromagnetic field. His body began alerting the immune system with the very first exposure when he ate the fruit at lunch in the airplane. That was the first exposure. Sitting near the melon for hours was the second and third exposure, all in one day. His immune system couldn't take it anymore and it did what it was supposed to do.

I rushed to the kitchen. My husband was about to dial 911.

"Wait for a second." I told him in a hurried voice. " I think he is reacting to the watermelon. Let's treat him and see if he will respond to NAET before we call 911."

I grabbed a knife, cut a piece of watermelon, put it in a glass jar and reached Ravi's bedside, all in a few seconds. Unlike my husband, I am very quick and spontaneous in doing things. I am always hyperactive and never knew the word "relax." In the room I threw the pillows down and made Ravi hold the glass jar and gave him an NAET treatment, all done in a few seconds to a minute. I didn't have time to explain anything. He was sitting there helplessly struggling to catch his breath. His wife stood there staring at me, watching me work on him. She was scared and paralyzed with fear. Sina was a simple housewife from a remote village in India.

It took approximately a minute to complete the NAET back treatment. Soon after I completed the back treatment, I looked at Ravi's face. He was breathing easier. The whistling became less noisy and eventually faded away. I watched the sweat beads drying away on his forehead and face, as the color returned. In less than five minutes, he was breathing normally again.

"What was that about?" he asked, staring at me with wide

eyes filled with surprise.

"How do you feel now, Ravi?" I inquired.

"I am feeling better." He smiled and replied. "For a minute I thought I was close to my end. I was so afraid and mainly afraid for her," he pointed towards Sina. "Thank God you were able to help me. I never had anything like this before."

"That is the new treatment she had discovered last year to treat allergies," my husband said. "It works well with any kind of allergies to reduce the symptoms quickly."

"Wow!," he exclaimed. "It worked like magic!."

"She thought you had an allergy to watermelon and that caused your breathing problem." Kris explained. " She just treated you for an allergy to watermelon."

"Whatever she did, I am so grateful to her," said Ravi. "It is very scary when you can't get your breath. My maternal uncle had asthma and he died from it when he was just 32."

"Did you ever have asthma, Ravi?" I asked.

"Never." He said. "I suffered from constant cough and bronchitis while growing up. I was repeatedly taking antibiotics until I was fifteen or so. Then I started running. I was an inter-school champion in running. Ever since I started running, my bronchitis and cough stopped."

I had to repeat NAET on him one more time after fifteen minutes. Then he went to sleep. When he woke up at 6:00 a.m., he looked fine. When he was leaving for the airport, he whispered, "Thank you, my lifesaver!"

I smiled. But in my heart I was trying to find appropriate

words to thank God for helping me to help Ravi with that unexpected emergency.

That was the first time I realized that NAET could also help with asthma.

Ravi and Sina were amazing. They kept telling everyone their story and told them that I had discovered a new instant cure for asthma. Within the next few months, family friends and their friends flew to LA from different parts of the country to get treated for their asthma. Most of them lived in my house while going through the treatments. I gave two treatments a day and they didn't mind to eat just white rice and cauliflower for the entire stay. Some stayed one week and some two weeks. But each one of them felt much better before they left, and they all returned for two weeks at a time for a few more times until they completed the program. They all got complete freedom from their asthma when they completed the whole NAET program.

I then incorporated NAET treatments for asthma into my practice. I have treated many hundreds of asthmatic patients, with excellent results. Asthma is curable—100% curable. One needs to understand the pathophysiology of asthma which can be understood through Oriental medical theory. Once one understands the cause, identifies the allergen, detects the mode of entry, NAET treatments are capable of removing the allergic affinity of your body with the allergen permanently. Everyone is different. Allergens affect everyone differently. So the treatments should be designed accordingly. Western medical researchers are still looking for the causes that trigger asthma. They are getting frustrated by not finding any reportable cause. Oriental medicine has simple answers that will help the medical practitioners help their patients effectively, to reduce the asthmatic symptoms and, if combined with NAET, the reactions to the desensitized item can be eliminated permanently.

NAET believes that almost all health problems begin with some allergies. If one can learn to detect the allergens one can stay away from the allergens. Just by staying away might help a person live a normal life. The technique to test and find your own allergies is described in Chapter 6. One has to be a medically trained person to learn the treatments. Teaching the treatments is beyond the scope of this book. Once you detect your allergens, either avoid them or find an NAET practitioner near you and get a series of treatments. I have trained over 7000 medical practitioners all over the world. Most of their names and addresses can be obtained by visiting our web site, "www.naet.com."

Devi S. Nambudripad
M.D., D.C., L.Ac., Ph.D. (Acu.).
January, 2004

INTRODUCTION

It is your *human right* to eat whatever food you like to eat, live in whatever environment you like, wear what ever clothes or cosmetics you want, live with whomever you prefer, and be able to breathe normally. If you are not able to accomplish this, you may be suffering from asthma or some other respiratory disorder.

People without having first-hand knowledge of NAET might get confused by the above statement.

People have been suffering from asthma for a long time, probably from the beginning of the human existence. No one knows the cause of this disorder. So everyone treats the symptoms by observing the signs and symptoms of this disorder. In other words, we have symptom-oriented treatments. NAET theory believes that some software problems (a Virus perhaps?) in the brain-computer is the cause of asthma and asthma-related illnesses. Some people may have this software problem from the time they are born or some may have acquired it during this lifetime. NAET testing procedures can help you understand the underlying cause of your asthma.

NAET is a way to reprogram one's brain to its original state. NAET is the computer virus treatment to help one's brain to remove the faulty program and replace with the correct one.

NAET is not a magic cure for anything. I don't want readers to get any wrong idea by reading this book. It is pure hard work. Hard work based on stone-hard Oriental healing arts. If you are not willing to work hard, if you expect a magic bullet to cure all your problems, NAET is not for you. If you are willing to work hard, willing to make changes in your life-style, you can get relief of asthma or any asthma-related medical symptoms I have mentioned anywhere in this book or in any of my other books. I have treated every one of those allergy-based problems successfully with NAET. If they are not allergies or originating from allergies, NAET is not the way to go.

The main application of NAET is to remove the adverse reactions between your body and other substances and thus to provide you with good nutrition, and enhance your natural ability to absorb, assimilate the necessary elements from your food and eliminate the unwanted and toxic materials when they get into your body by any means. NAET advises you to test everything around you for possible allergies before you put it in your mouth or apply on your body or bring it close to your body (electromagnetic field). If you are allergic to every ingredient in your diet, no matter how pure and clean your diet is, you will never find a single healthy day in your life. If you are allergic to your own digestive juices [stomach acid (HCL) and digestive enzymes or base], no matter what simple food you eat, no matter what high quality digestive enzymes you take, you will have indigestion (bloating, flatulence, sensation of heaviness, brain fog, overweight, underweight, heaviness in the head, poor elimination, etc.) and any of these can lead to asthma. One can be allergic to environments: grasses, weeds, flowers, bees, insects, etc. which are supposed to create a clean environment, and if you are allergic to them you could never step out of your room without getting asthma. If you are allergic to pesticides (pesticides are loaded with heavy metals, mercury, etc.) and other environmental toxins, again you may have to be shut in.

How can you hide from all these and live? When you get treated with NAET, your body will not react to these allergens anymore. When you get them into your body, the body will throw them out through natural elimination processes without alerting the immune system. As long as you are allergic to these, your body will alert the immune system every time they come near you and trigger an asthma attack. After you replace the faulty program with a new, corrected one by treating and clearing the allergies to nutritious foods and products, you will be able to consume them freely without getting sick.

If you check around, you will realize 95% of human illnesses originate from some form of allergies. So the real cause of your asthma is allergy. The virus in the brain's software causes a programming error and this causes inappropriate responses to every allergic stimuli coming into the body. Many people think mercury, pesticides, environmental toxins, etc. cause asthma or other respiratory disorders. In my opinion, one's allergic tendency (programming error) makes one react to these toxins and causes such serious illnesses. After successful NAET treatment program for these toxins, we are finding reversal of such problems.

One might argue that the people who do not react adversely to the above toxins have good immune systems. Yes, I do agree. But how did they get good immune systems? Good immunity either inherited or they have no allergy to the pesticides, environmental toxins or chemicals. Again the allergy is the underlying cause—whether it is a reaction to chemicals or environmental toxins. Many of my asthma patients are doing well after they were desensitized to these toxins through NAET.

If the doctors and patients learn to use NAET testing techniques (read Chapter 6), and treatments, we can put an end to allergy-related asthma and other lung disorders.

NAET stresses the importance of life-style changes. Consuming non-allergic food and drinks, living in a non-allergic environment, using non-allergic chemicals, associating with non allergic people, getting adequate exercise, all this means life-style changes. It means giving up eating junk food, and drinking non-nutritious sodas, giving up refined sugars and alcohol and eating more vegetables, and wholesome nutritious foods.

Some people may get scared of that regimen. But I have news for you. When you complete the NAET treatments successfully —

(I stress on this: *complete the treatment successfully*— because I have come to know that some practitioners are not doing NAET properly and they are mixing NAET with other treatments and not getting the expected result from NAET treatments), you stop craving wrong things. Your body will begin craving more meaningful items like fresh vegetables, wholesome foods, etc. instead of junk foods. If you are a sugar addict before NAET, after completing treatments, you will give up eating sugar and you would not even miss it. That has been our experience for the past 20 years. You will become health-oriented naturally.

NAET will guide you in the right direction, will give you an opportunity to work hard and lead a normal life. Most people with asthma live in fear. They are afraid to go out of their comfort zones, they are afraid to travel, or eat at a regular restaurant for fear of reactions. You are advised to eat limited foods during the treatment phase, but after the 25-hours of each treatment, you should eat non-allergic, wholesome foods to receive adequate nutrition. After successful completion of allergy treatment you won't react much to foods and environments. Once in a while if you eat at McDonald's or Taco Bell, your body will not collapse. You will be able to handle it with ease. This is a 21st Century treatment. You will be free to live in this world again. Eating refined foods and junk food can put more stress on your system without giving you any benefit of nutrients. You need to live sensibly. Moderation of everything at every level is the key to long-term good health.

Say Good-bye to Asthma will help you understand your illness and will assist you in finding the right help to achieve better health.

Say Good-bye to Asthma will show you how certain commonly used products can trigger asthma; how such problems have a domino effect that can end in serious complications; how your problems can relate to allergy, a traditionally under-diagnosed or misdiagnosed condition; and, how allergies can manifest into myriad lung symptoms that might seem unrelated.

It's not enough to treat symptoms with medication or a piecemeal therapy. These usually just put a "bandage" on the sore, so to speak. *Say Good-bye to Asthma* gets to the root of health problems and will help you in eliminating their reactions.

This book will show you how you can find help to reprogram your brain (central nervous system) to accept all foods, chemicals, environmental factors, and products as neutral or beneficial– although not in one session. You may need many sessions with your practitioner or do it yourself if you have many mild or hidden allergies. You will learn how allergy might have caused your asthma. You will learn how genetic allergies and allergy-related illness can now be controlled.

Your brain is an obliging organ that has been searching for ways to help you feel better through much trial and error and various levels of homeostasis (balance). Now it can do the job it has been trying to do. Through NAET, your reprogrammed brain will have learned to accept substances it previously rejected and will allow your body to react normally to the elements of your life so you can get on your way to perfect health.

NAET was developed by Dr. Devi S. Nambudripad, who has been treating asthma patients with this technique since 1985, and teaching other health professionals how to administer it since 1989. To date, more than 7,000 licensed medical practitioners have been trained in NAET procedures and are practicing all over the world. For more information on NAET or for an NAET practitioner near you, log on to the NAET website: www.naet.com.

Who Should Use This Book?

Anyone who is suffering from asthma or suffering from an allergy-related disease or condition should read this book. This natural, non invasive technique is ideal to treat infants, children, grown-ups, old and debilitated people who suffer from mild to severe allergic reactions without altering their current plan of treatment. NAET encourages the use of all medications, supplements or other therapies while going through the NAET program. When the patient gets better, the patient's regular physician can reduce or alter the dosage of drugs.

How is This Book Organized?

Chapter 1-Explains asthma and allergies in general terms.

Chapter 2-Describes the effects of inhalant allergens.

Chapter 3-Describes the categories of all other allergens.

Chapter 4-Explains Nambudripad's Testing Techniques and gives you information on various other allergy testing techniques.

Chapter 5- Explains more on asthma assessment.

Chapter 6-Explains NMST(NeuroMuscular Sensitivity testing) to detect allergies.

Chapter 7-Discusses the pathological symptoms of acupuncture meridians.

Chapter 8-Describes NAET Allergens.

Chapter 9-Describes self-balancing techniques.

Chapter 10-Discusses allergies, nutrition, and exercise.

Glossary- This section will help you to understand the appropriate meaning of the medical terminology used in this book.

Resources-Provided to assist you in finding natural products and consultants to support you while you work with your allergies.

Bibliography- Since NAET is an energy balancing treatment, supporting bibliography on this subject is hard to find. This book cannot be completed without mentioning valuable information on Oriental Medicine and acupuncture, because NAET was developed from Oriental Medicine. Since NAET uses basic information from allopathy, kinesiology and chiropractic, books explaining these subject are also given in the bibliography.

Index- A detailed index is included to help you locate your area of interest quickly and easily.

Looking for Real Causes of Your Illness?

Anyone who is desperate to find "REAL CAUSES" for his/her allergies or illnesses after experiencing many disappointing trials and tribulations for long time, should read this book with open mind and heart ready to learn about NAET which will definitely guide you to the road of Healing.

Dr. Nambudripad has utililzed all her skills as Chiropractor, Acupuncturist, Oriental and Allopathic M.D., to author and practice NAET since 1980's and has helped numerous patients back to health without burdening the patients to financial ruin. Her compassion and empathy for the sick and uncompromising character contribute so much to her practice of NAET. As a Medical Doctor trained in allopathic medicine and practiced for over 16 years, I have learned by reading the book and practicing, NAET is the most impotant tool in Healing the whole person. All the healthcare professionals who are disappointed and tired of practicing "symptomatic treatments" and dealing with the side-effects with more "symptomatic treatments," should definitely read this book. If you are not blinded by the bias and prejudice of your own profession and the healthcare Industries, the book will open your eyes and heart to learn that NAET is an incredibly powerful tool to detect the causes of asthma and other allergy-related illnesses and therefore treat the disease naturally and effectively. Practicing NAET will bring back the "Passion" that we had once as we joined the healthcare career to "help the suffering," and your patients will love you for being a true "Healer."

Lisa Camerino, M.D.
Portland, Oregon

1

About Asthma

Asthma is one of the world's most common health problems. The World Health Organization estimates that asthma affects nearly 150 million people worldwide. In the United States, asthma affects 14 to 15 million people. Among the reported cases, it is one of the leading causes of school and work absences and the most common chronic disease of childhood.

The word asthma comes from the Greek, meaning "I gasp for breath." It was used by Hippocrates (460-370 B.C.) to denote certain types of breathing difficulties.

Asthma is an allergic state in which the bronchial tubes constrict the passage of air, resulting in severe difficulty breathing and a whistling type of exhalation. The sides of the airways in the lungs become thick and swollen, causing recurring episodes of wheezing, breathlessness, tightness and aching of the chest, and throat constriction-like sensations. Sufferers often have a persistent cough that lasts more than a week or coughing attacks after laughing, crying, brisk-walking, or exercising. Some people wake up in the middle of night coughing or wheezing, especially between 3 a.m. and 5 a.m, the lung meridian time (See Chapter 7).

If not halted in the initial stages, asthma can become a chronic inflammatory disease of the airways. Attacks occur spasmodically but can be severe at times. The sensation of suffocation can be so severe that a person feels he/she is choking to death. In some cases, an attack of asthma does prove fatal.

Many thousands of people in every part of the world who suffer from asthma have been unable to find relief or appropriate medical help for various reasons.

Breathing is the first bodily function which starts at birth and remains the most essential function of life until death. All living beings are bestowed with one free thing in this world – the air to breathe. Breathing is everyone's birthright. Unfortunately for some people, the respiratory system becomes dysfunctional, affected by the various ongoing physical and mental abuses of everyday life.

But life must go on... so the person with poor respiratory health must move forward huffing and puffing, struggling to get air into and out of the lungs, not knowing the cause of the malady.

Now, with *Say Good-bye to Asthma* and NAET, relief is in sight.

What is NAET?

Nambudripad's Allergy Elimination Technique (NAET) is a natural, painless, and noninvasive treatment used in desensitization, reduction, or permanent elimination of various food, chemical and environmental allergies. Most asthma and lung disorders are caused from allergies.

NAET utilizes Oriental medical diagnostic procedures exclusively for diagnosing and treating asthma and allergies. But NAET uses other standard diagnostic procedures and standard allergy testing procedures from allopathy, kinesiology, and chiropractic (Read Chapter 4), and an electrodermal computerized allergy testing procedure to support the NAET diagnosis done through Oriental Medical procedures.

This treatment does not involve the use of drugs, herbs, vitamins, or other supplements. However, NAET may be used in conjunction with other forms of treatments and therapies including drugs, herbs, vitamins, minerals, other supplements or thera-

ASTHMA?

Elimination of Asthma?!? Is it possible?" I asked when I first heard about Dr. Devi and NAET. "Absolutely!" is the answer to that question I later discovered after meeting Devi and learning her amazingly simple, most effective technique. Bar none, no other allergy treatment in my practice has been as effective as NAET. Dr. Devi is truly a medical pioneer, and she has my deepest respect, both personally and professionally. TELL EVERYONE YOU KNOW about the best-kept secret in the world of allergy and asthma diagnosis and therapy: NAET.

NAET Sp: Ann McCombs, D.O.
Medical Director
Center for Optimum Health
Seattle, Washington
(425) 576- 0951

pies, if they are found appropriate to improve or enhance your health. Each item, however, should be tested and cleared for any possible allergy before using.

THE MEDICAL I CHING

NAET uses a testing procedure called *The Medical I Ching* (pronounced as Eee Cheeng) from Oriental Medical testing procedures. The *I Ching* or Classic of change is the essence of Chinese philosophy. In China, this *I Ching* has been revered as the most profound book of wisdom. Without the principles of *yin and yang of the I Ching,* one cannot even envisage Oriental philosophy. According to Chinese tradition, *I Ching* was developed by Fu Xi, the most ancient Chinese culture hero in 3,322 BC. Journeying through the past 6,000 years, I Ching has passed through many generations. Numerous variations of original *I Ching* have been born and practiced by various medical professionals everywhere.

MUSCLE RESPONSE TESTING

Kinesiological muscle response testing is a variation of Chinese *I Ching.* Muscle response testing has been practiced in this country since 1964. In this country, it was originated by Dr. George Goodheart and his associates. Dr. John F. Thie advocates this method through the "Touch For Health" Foundation in Malibu, California. Interested readers can write to "Touch For Health" Foundation for information and books on the subject.

NEURO MUSCULAR SENSITIVITY TESTING

NMST (Neuro Muscular Sensitivity Testing), another variation of *I Ching*, is practiced by NAET specialists. Even though NMST appears to be similar to kinesiological muscle response testing, it is slightly different from regular kinesiological muscle response testing procedure from its concept and application.

If used properly, NMST has the unique ability to retrieve information from your autonomic nervous system (sympathetic and parasympathetic nervous systems) about most stages of your health problems (mild, moderate or severe symptoms).

NAET also utilizes other Oriental medical principles and procedures to evaluate your health status by detecting energy blockages in acupuncture meridians.

NAET evaluates the status of the compatibility of daily consumed food, drinks, supplements to trace the cause of your asthma and other respiratory discomforts. NAET emphasizes correct nutrition to get the best results and control your asthma symptoms. You are what you eat! If you are allergic to what you eat, then food, for you, becomes an allergen and your health suffers. But foods are not the only possible allergens.

To accomplish allergy elimination, NAET utilizes a combination of kinesiology, acupuncture, acupressure, nutritional management and a specific type of gentle, spinal manipulative procedure derived from chiropractic methods.

The secret to good health is achieved through correct nutrition.

WHAT IS CORRECT NUTRITION?

Correct or right nutrition does not mean buying expensive food, drinks or supplements. It means non-allergic foods, drinks and supplements.

THE MAIN GOAL

The principal goal of this book is to reach out to all asthma sufferers, to educate about your asthmatic reactions, to help remove confusion and idiosyncrasies about treatment procedures, and to provide guidance for you to achieve better health.

This book provides unique, useful information to evaluate this life-threatening condition from a different perspective than standard medical evaluations. In this book you will find various self-tests to detect asthma and asthma-related conditions before they become chronic. If you discover the signs and symptoms, however mild they may be in the initial stages, you are advised to seek appropriate help immediately. Seeking timely help before the condition manifests fully will assist in full recovery.

TREATMENT FOR ASTHMA

This book is not intended to teach you to self-treat asthma. That is beyond its scope. Asthma is a serious condition. It should be treated by a well-qualified, experienced medical professional. But this book will guide you to understand this condition and how a very effective, alternate testing technique can be used to detect the causes (Read Chapter 6). As obvious as that sounds, please be aware that many health professionals do not look for or find causes; they treat symptoms. Once causes are determined and eliminated by reprogramming the brain, asthma can often be eradicated permanently. NAET techniques are designed to do just that.

Different ethnic heritage and socioeconomic conditions greatly affect respiratory disorders and asthma. Let's look at some of the published statistics on these issues:

According to a report from CDC, between 1980 and 1995, the percentage of children with asthma doubled, rising from 3.6 percent in 1980 to 7.5 percent in 1995. A decrease in the percentage of children with asthma occurred between 1995 and 1996, but interpreting single-year changes is difficult.

The percentage of children with asthma differs by race, ethnicity and socioeconomic factors. In 1997- 2000, more than 8 percent of Black non-Hispanic children living in families with incomes below the poverty level had an asthma attack in the previous 12 months. Approximately 6 percent of White non-Hispanic children and 5 percent of Hispanic children living in families with incomes below the poverty level had an asthma attack in the previous 12 months. Emergency room visits for asthma and other respiratory causes were 369 per 10,000 children in 1992 and 379 per 10,000 children in 1999. Hospital admissions for asthma and other respiratory causes were 55 per 10,000 children in 1980 and 66 per 10,000 children in 1999.

According to one survey, 94% of sufferers reported that they suffered from asthma for a long time and that asthma reduced their quality of life. Even though many knew that they suffered from asthma, they didn't take the diagnosis too seriously and suffered the consequences. They left their health to destiny and didn't do anything about it. About 50% of people with the problem consider the disease a serious medical condition, but less than a third consulted a medical practitioner or an allergist.

Asthma sufferers have trouble getting a good night's sleep, engaging in outdoor activities, being able to concentrate, being productive at work, and enjoying a satisfying family life. People with asthma or with the family history of asthma should have a complete check up by a qualified medical practitioner and should take measures to curtail asthma immediately.

CAUSES OF ASTHMA

- Disruption of the brain's "software program" is the main cause of allergies and illness. Asthma is not any different from other illnesses. The brain's computer software can have the equivalent of a virus or, in some cases, many viruses collected during a person's life or transferred to the person through the genes from parents and grandparents. These viruses cause malfunction of the software; in turn the related vital organ-functions are disrupted. In the case of asthma, respiratory functions are disrupted. This causes the lungs and respiratory tract to become sensitive to aspects of the person's environment. The malfunctioning program no longer recognizes things around the body without appropriate reprogramming. These software "viruses" may have found their entry into the body through the following routes:

- Heredity: This is the most important factor in the case of asthma. An allergic tendency is inherited from parents and family as dominant or recessive, but allergic manifestation may vary from generation to generation. For example, if a parent suffered from migraines, eczema or arthritis, offspring may suffer from asthma – not necessarily experiencing the exact manifestation of parents or other family members. In severe, stubborn cases of asthma it is often seen that genetic characteristics from various ancestors or generations have been accumulated and transmitted to the offspring and the child suffers the cumulative effect of the inheritance as an extremely severe manifestation of asthma.

- Toxins: Food allergy toxins cause asthma in many people. For example, toxins from foods and food proteins such as egg, milk, casein, albumin, peanuts, wheat, fish, soy and other legumes.

- Toxins from food additives and food preservatives: Various food additives are used to preserve the texture, color and shelf-life of prepackaged or pre-made foods. Some of the commonly used additives are as follows: Acetic acid, agar, aldicarb, alginates, aluminum salts, corn products, carob, propylene glycol, sodium aluminum phosphates, benzoates, calcium proprionate, calcium silicate, carbamates, ethylene gas, food bleach, formic acid, malic acid, mannan, M.S.G., salicylic acid, succinic acid, sulfites, talc, and tartaric acid.

- Food colorings: Yellow and red dyes, soft drinks, margarine, orange drinks, cheese, cakes, cookies, candies, crackers, ice creams, and syrups.

- Medications: Prescription or nonprescription drugs, aspirins or aspirin products, over-the-counter pain relievers, antacids, vitamin supplements, herbal supplements and nutritional supplements or replacements like protein drinks, etc.

- Molds and fungi: Stale breads, stale prepared foods (food leftovers more than 24 hours old), cakes, yeast products, airborne spores, mushrooms, etc.

- Latex products: Plastic products, crude oil products, synthetic materials, dry cleaning chemicals, fabrics, wool, animal dander, and epithelials.

- Dust mites: House-dust, industrial dust, insects.

- Inhalants/irritants: Pollens, grasses, weeds, other environmental agents, animal epithelial, animal dander, pesticides, house cleaning chemicals, chemically treated city water, drinking water, industrial waste, polluted air, smoke, cigarette smoke, smell from cooking gas, cooking, seasoning, frying, spicy foods, gas burning, smoke from fireplace, wood burning, barbecuing, wildfire burning, smoke from volcano, perfume, liquid propane, carbon monoxide, carbon dioxide, fluorocarbons in hair sprays, cleaning sprays, smell from animals, smell of various body secretions from self and others (stool, urine, sputum, sweat, bad breath), flowers, chemical smells, smell from fabrics, etc.

- Infections: Toxins produced in the body from invasions of microorganisms such as virus, bacteria, parasite, yeast, etc., and mold, fungus, candida, ticks, etc.

- Building materials: Formaldehyde, paints, pressed wood, sheet rock, particle board, plywood, wood cabinets, side tables, end tables, furniture, bed, headboard, carpets, glues, etc.

- Vaccinations and immunizations.

- A depressed immune system due to chronic illnesses, autoimmune disorders, etc.

- Malabsorption disorders: Nutritional deficiencies, digestive problems, poor absorption and assimilation of nutrients due to an allergy to the nutrients, eating overcooked, infected, or unsuitable food or the unavailability of food.

- Hormonal deficiencies: Removal of reproductive organs, dysfunction of ovaries, thyroid glands, hypothalamus, deficiency of female and male hormones, adrenal and pituitary hormones.

- Posttraumatic disorders: Surgery, accidents, delivery, stressful work, school, life-style, war veterans, etc.

- Gastric reflux disorders: Hyperacidity, reflux disease, etc.

- Radiation and geopathic stress: Working long hours with computers, allergy to computer radiation, sitting in front of televisions, living near or under powerful electrical cables, living near power plants, exposure to radioactive materials, working under extreme weather conditions without proper clothing.

- Poor physical activity: Small-scale toxins produced in the body from minor reactions and interactions will flush out naturally if one maintains good physical activities.
- Emotional traumas: Disharmony of mind-body-spirit due to traumas from past or present, childhood abuses, abuses and traumas in other ages, troubled emotions like chronic fear, anger, cult association, victimization, etc.

An allergic tendency toward asthma is inherited. Since it occurs much more frequently in families that have a history of various allergic conditions, the tendency toward this particular allergic ailment seems to be more frequently inherited than most other allergic diseases.

HOW TO CONTROL ASTHMA

Like other allergic conditions, asthma responds very well to NAET. It can reprogram the brain's *software* program to its original state or let's say "debug" it. NAET can erase the corrupted program and reinput the corrected data in your brain's computer.

When beginning NAET treatment, it is always better to combine Western medical treatments with NAET for better and faster results. After you are treated for the NAET Basic 15-30 groups, your asthma doctor can evaluate your symptoms and try to gradually reduce or adjust the dosage of any medication that you may be taking.

Asthma is not only a dangerous and distressing malady, but it also interferes with a person's ability to lead a normal life. If you suffer from asthma, you should receive prompt treatment. Asthmatics should always carry inhalant sprays for quick relief in emergencies because an asthmatic attack can be triggered at any time from a contact with an unexpected allergen.

Once I treated a student pediatric nurse who suffered from severe asthma from smelling fecal matter. Initially she began asthma symptoms while rotating in the pediatric floor as a nursing student by smelling fecal matter from infants and children. She was not able to identify the source of her asthma then and lived with asthma medication and sprays but continued to work in the pediatric ward after graduation. In the beginning, she noticed her asthma triggering only at work. When she left work, she felt better. Eventually, she began getting asthma symptoms upon arising in the morning too. Her asthma was getting progressively worse in spite of medication when she decided to seek some alternative help and was led to my office.

In my office during NMST (explained in Chapter 6), she was found to be reacting to the smell of fecal matter. When she was asked to trace back the first asthma occurrence, she was able to remember the first attack in the pediatric ward while she was a student. The initial cause was left untreated (medication only masks the symptoms, does not eliminate the cause), the problem got accentuated and eventually any bad smell began triggering asthma. She was successfully treated with NAET and she now lives a normal life.

Asthma usually first appears in infancy or childhood. However, onset of symptoms can occur at any age or, in some cases, reappear after many years of inactivity. The age of onset of an asthma condition depends on the degree of inheritance. The stronger the genetic factor, the earlier in life the onset.

People suffer from allergic manifestation in varying degrees because of different levels of parental inheritance. But regardless of age, gender, race, or inheritance, anyone can manifest allergies at any time if the tendency is present.

In some cases, even when parents had no allergies, their offspring might carry the genetic possibility for allergy. In these cases, various possibilities exist:

- Parents may have suffered from a serious disease or condition. Example: Malaria contracted before the child was born causing alteration in the genetic codes.
- Expectant mother may have been exposed to harmful substances like radiation (X-ray), chemicals, too much caffeine, alcohol, drugs or antibiotics.
- Toxins could have caused genetic mutation as the result of a disease (streptococcal infection as in strep-throat, measles or chicken pox).
- Pregnant mother may have suffered severe emotional trauma(s): Abuse, divorce, abandonment, death of the spouse, etc.
- Parents may have suffered severe malnutrition (not only not getting enough food, but not assimilating due to poor absorption or allergies), possibly causing the growing embryo to undergo cell mutation.

Any of these may cause alteration of the genetic codes for messages to be carried over to the next generation. The result–the organs and tissues that are supposed to develop normally may have impaired function.

In sensitive individuals, contact with any allergen can produce a variety of symptoms, in varying degrees ranging from mild itching to severe swelling of the tissues, or mild fatigue to severe anaphylaxis. The ingested, inhaled or contacted allergen is capable of alerting the immune system of the body. The frightened and confused immune system then commands the production and immediate release of immunoglobulins and other chemical mediators.

These immune system mediators are released as part of the body's immune response in order to counteract the effect of the invading foreign substances (allergens). Some people may be allergic to their own immune system mediators. In these sensitive people, their endogenous secretions or their immune system mediators produce abnormal physical, physiological and psychological symptoms in varying degrees when these chemicals are released into the blood stream to fight what the body considers dangerous invaders. When the body reacts adversely to immune mediators, the body loses the fight to the invader. Then the weak body exaggerates the physical, physiological or emotional response toward the invader, which then causes disease.

There are millions of potential allergens. Our bodies interact and react with them hundreds of times every day. Only some people react adversely where others live happily among them, enjoying their benefits. These "normal" people have normal immune systems. They did not inherit misinformed genes from their ancestors. When the immune system is working properly, allergic reactions are kept under control. A normal body releases appropriate immune system mediators to fight the invader and win. These mediators bring the situation under control in seconds by enhancing body functions to speed up the metabolic functions: neutralize the toxin or enhance the digestion in case the attacker is a food-protein, as in peanut; neutralize the chemical reaction in case the invader is pesticide, mercury, or a swimming pool chemical; destroy the toxin in case the attacker is bacteria, virus, or a parasite, etc.

In allergy-prone people, the normal imprint of a memory about the harmlessness of substances such as peanut, fish, pollen, dust, perfume, etc., has somehow been erased from the brain's memory due to certain stresses of life, most likely during the genetic transference. Some of these stresses of life may have happened due to the following reasons: Exposure to extreme radiation, bacterial toxins, toxins from exposure to heavy metals, or chemicals. This altered memory has substituted the original memory with new information that identifies the substance as being dangerous. Thus, the immune system mistakes a harmless substance for a dangerous intruder it must destroy. When a person with allergies is exposed to something it perceives to be an allergen, the immune system produces antibodies to fight it as a harmful invader.

What began as an innocent case of mistaken identity is now an allergic reaction possibly causing death if there is a complete shutdown of the system.

According to statistics released by CDC (Center for Disease control and AAAAI), more than 50 million Americans suffer from allergic diseases every year. Up to two million, or 8 percent, of children in the United States are estimated to be affected by food allergy. Up to 2 percent of adults are so affected. According to the CDC (1996 statistics), chronic sinusitis is the most commonly reported chronic disease, affecting 12.6 percent of people (approximately 38 million). According to the Journal of the American Medical Association (270:2456-63, 1993), allergy to the venom of stinging insects (honeybees, wasps, hornets, yellow jackets, and fire ants) is relatively common, with prevalence of systemic reactions in American adults of 3.3 percent. The Journal of Allergy and Clinical Immunology (103:559-62, 1999) reported that peanut or tree nut allergies affect approximately 3 million Americans and cause the most severe food-induced allergic reactions. AAAAI reported that seasonal allergic rhinitis, often referred to as "hay fever," affects more than 35 million people in the United States. According to the statistical report from AAAAI, if one parent has allergic disease, the estimated risk of a child developing allergies is 48 percent; the child's estimated risk grows to 70 percent if both parents have a history of allergy.

Some of the common allergy-based disorders are:

- Sneezing
- Stuffy or runny nose
- Coughing
- Watery or itchy eyes
- Itchy throat and nose
- Postnasal drip
- Itchy skin or rash
- Hives
- Allergies may also cause unfamiliar reactions. These may include:
- Conjunctivitis (red eye)
- Dark circles under the eyes (AKA "allergic shiners")
- Stomach cramps, anxiety, or shortness of breath in anaphylaxis cases
- Seasonal rhinitis, perennial rhinitis
- Emotional reactions like anger and fear

Many allergy and asthma sufferers struggle silently without knowing how to regain their birthright that was lost due to living in this polluted, contaminated, complicated, world.

There are various reasons why certain silent sufferers continue the struggle to breathe or refuse to seek help. I have come across many different types of asthma victims during my 20 years of practice. When you read through the list below, you might recognize many of them.

1. Most of the unfortunate asthma victims do not know they suffer from asthma. They know they have something wrong with them but never thought it was asthma.

2. Some of them are aware of it but they do not have any medical facility available near them.

3. Some of them are aware of it but cannot afford to see a doctor due to lack of funds. Medical help is costly.

4. Some of them cannot afford time off from their busy schedules to visit a doctor or medical facility.

5. Some others are depressed because of their health conditions, and have no energy to seek medical help to solve their breathing problem.

6. Some others refuse to get medical help because they want to punish their family and friends by forcing them to watch the victim struggle to breathe.

7. Some of them refuse to take treatments even if the treatments are available to them because if they get better they do not get attention from their loved ones.

8. Some people refuse to admit that they have any health problem and refuse to get help from any medical discipline.

9. Some others dislike doctors (from any medical discipline) and refuse to seek help from them.

10. Some people like to suffer the maximum in this life so that they will be rewarded in another life.

11. Some people do not want to get better because they do not want to go back to their previous life-style because the purpose of living is changed now (divorce, death, loss of job, etc.).

12. Some refuse to seek help because "God" gave them asthma and God will be upset if they got treatment without His approval and do not know how to get His approval in this life.

The fact is that there are very few human diseases or conditions in which allergic factors are not involved either directly or indirectly. Any substance under the sun, including sunlight itself, can cause an allergic reaction in sensitive individuals.

Avoidance is the best solution Western medicine can offer to prevent asthma and allergies. Even with avoidance, there is no guarantee that asthma sufferers will be able to stay away from every situation and still remain reaction free. With the progress of science and technology, our modern life-styles have changed dramatically. New products, which are potential allergens for many people, are being developed every day. The quality of life has improved; but for some allergic patients, scientific achievements have merely created more nightmares.

We are living in the twenty-first century where technology is predominant. There is nothing wrong with the technology. Modern technology has provided a better quality of life. But in order to enjoy life, the asthma patient must find ways to overcome adverse reactions to drugs, chemicals and other allergens produced by technology.

Of course, in America, you have access to many hundreds of lifesaving, miraculous, pharmaceutical products for helping with asthma and allergy victims. If your asthma is not due to an allergy, or if you are not allergic to the drugs you are taking, then you can get appropriate drugs and take them to control your asthma or other allergic disorders with satisfaction. But what will be your outcome if you are allergic to the medication that is supposed to help you? Even though drugs are enormously expensive, here in America, you also have various means to purchase them and use them. If one medicine did not work, you have the opportunity to use another one, if that didn't work, yet another one, until you find the right one to help you in your need.

THE UNIVERSAL PROBLEM

But Asthma is a UNIVERSAL problem. Many millions suffer from asthma in other less privileged countries. Some fortunate people there have money for their medication; the rest suffer silently, or leave their health to destiny to decide upon. They have no access to get one square meal a day let alone the medicine.

NAET has strict rules of food restrictions and avoidance while going through the treatment. Even though it is only for 25 hours at a time, many modern-day people do not want to inconvenience themselves to go through such strict regimen either due to their life-style or work schedule. There are very effective drugs for such people. They just need to find the right one.

But NAET may the best solution for other people, with allergies to drugs, and people who live in third world countries or in less privileged countries.

O. M. THEORY ON ASTHMA

According to Oriental medical theory, asthma, allergies and allergy-based disorders are the results of long-term energy disturbances in the energy pathways (please read Chapter 7). Severe allergic reactions are caused by severe energy disturbance in more than one energy meridians.

TYPES OF ALLERGIC REACTIONS

There are two major types of reactions to allergens (may they be foods, environments, or chemicals). An allergic reaction to proteins from nuts, fish, etc. can cause an immediate reaction that may result in an immediate closure of the throat due to swelling, or cause sudden asthma, hives, rise in temperature over two degrees, excessive mucus production, etc. The second type is a delayed reaction. This may cause symptoms in varying intensities (mild, moderate or severe but not extremely severe) on the same day or the next day or even days later; for examples, mild, occasional cough, mild wheezing, poor clarity in thinking, absent mindedness, brain fog, dizziness, headaches, vertigo, insomnia, general fatigue, ear-nose-throat problems, walking pneumonia, bronchitis, sinusitis, postnasal drips, pain in the chest, backaches, sub acute infections, ear infections, indigestion, elimination problems, arthritis, other joint disorders, skin problems, dermatitis, eczema, rash, diarrhea, hair loss, weight gain, weight loss, emotional imbalances such as anger, depression, irritability, hyperactivity, mood swings, etc.

WESTERN MEDICINE

In Western medicine, we have no definite explanations to why reactions happen immediately in some people and delayed in others and what factors determine that specificity of reactions. Using currently available Western diagnostic procedures, we cannot explain the mode of entry or exit of an allergen, we do not have any means to explain when and how the reaction would happen in one's body.

ORIENTAL MEDICINE

Even though Oriental medicine is 4000 + year old, using Oriental medical diagnostic procedures, we are able to detect the mode of entry of the allergen into the body and what to expect from such entry. If the diagnosis is right, treatment is easier.

NAET offers the prospect of relief to those who suffer from asthma and allergies by reprogramming the brain to perfect health. Just like rebooting a computer, we can reboot our nervous system through NAET to overcome the adverse reactions of brain and body.

To *fully* understand NAET, one needs to know some Oriental medical principles since NAET is developed from Oriental medical theories and techniques among others. No other medical discipline understands the human body better. NAET has taken the acupuncture and Oriental medical theories and developed a technique that can eliminate the reaction from the root-cause. Some people might raise their eyebrows, and ask, "Can you really eliminate my allergy or asthma reactions?"

NAET answers with a resounding *yes*.

Western medicine does not have satisfactory answers to many of today's medical questions. But it has developed sophisticated, effective pharmacopia. If one understands Oriental medicine, combines it with NAET and with the best of what is available in Western medicine or other medical disciplines, you will find your freedom from asthma soon and not miss much fun in this world. We live only once. There is no fun in living in misery. Ill health is misery. Health is wealth and health is happiness. If you have health, you have everything. If you do not have health, no matter what else you have, everything will be useless. How well I know that! Because I have been in both places—without health and with health.

If one can evaluate an asthma patient and understand the asthma's origin beginning with Oriental medical principles, NAET can remove the problem. In some cases it may take just a few NAET treatments to remove your asthma, but others may take several office visits depending on other factors. In both cases there is nothing to lose... there is much to gain:

The freedom to breathe freely again!

2

Categories of Allergens Part-1

As mentioned in Chapter 1, asthma and many other illnesses are caused by disruption of the brain's "Software" program. As such, asthma is an allergic condition in which the lungs and respiratory tract have become sensitive to a person's environment. An allergen is a substance that induces an allergic reaction. An allergen can be one of the causes of asthma. Once causes are determined and treated by NAET, asthma can often be permanently eradicated.

Common allergens are generally classified into nine basic categories based primarily on the method in which they are contacted, rather than the symptoms they produce.

Basic Categories of Allergens

1. Inhalants
2. Ingestants
3. Contactants
4. Injectants
5. Infectants

6. Physical Agents

7. Genetic Factors

8. Molds and Fungi

9. Emotional Stressors

Inhalants

Inhalants are those allergens that are contacted through the nose, throat and bronchial tubes. Breathing can be hazardous if you are allergic to particles in the air. Aside from oxygen, the air contains a wide variety of particles from different sources.

The usual diseases that result from airborne allergens are:

- Hay fever
- Allergic rhinitis
- Asthma (different kinds)
- Conjunctivitis
- Sinusitis
- Bronchiolitis
- Bronchitis (acute and chronic)
- Emphysema
- Pneumonia (different kinds)
- Cough

The following allergens can trigger asthma and above mentioned respiratory systems disorders when inhaled by sensitive individuals.

NAET is truly awesome. You will want to pass this book on to others and spread the word about this amazing technique. Anyone who has wrestled with asthma and allergies and a rotation diet or tried to eliminate wheat, sugar, and dairy from daily diet for years knows what a struggle that can be. But with the NAET process all of this becomes unnecessary. An allergen can be eliminated within 25 hours of treatment! No more having to avoid the food. No need to live with asthma and other allergies for life. You can easily, painlessly eliminate your allergies and allergy symptoms like asthma go away with the allergens. By finding an NAET practitioner in your area, and following through with the treatments, you and your family can get a new lease on life and tackle new horizons.

NAET Sp: Sandra C. Denton, M.D.
Clinical Ecologist
Alaska Alternative Medical Center
Anchorage, Alaska
(907) 563-6200

• Microscopic spores of certain grasses, flowers, pollens, tree pollens (more severe in certain seasons), insecticides, fertilizers, flour from grains, powders and fine particles from dried leaves, flowers and other parts from plants,.

• Cooking smells, smells from coffee brewing, popcorn popping, perfumes, cosmetics, smoke from cigarettes and cigars, wood burning from fireplace, from barbecue, wildfire burning, chemical fumes (smells from paint, washing soaps, detergents, dry cleaning chemicals, household cleaning chemicals, swimming pool chemicals), smells from your own or other's body secretions (stool, urine, sweat, semen, menstrual blood, etc) and smell from stale foods, decayed materials from outside, etc.

- Dust, dust mites
- Animal proteins (dander, hair, skin, and/or discharges)
- Spores from mold and fungus
- Insect parts: cockroaches, flea, bee, fly, ants - dead or alive; any part can affect sensitive people.

It is difficult to say that there is a typical or predictable allergic reaction, or set of reactions, in response to a given allergen because each person is different. This makes absolute predictability impossible. If there is a predictable response, however, it is in this general category of inhalants that it comes closest to being found.

Most of us have suffered the discomfort that comes from accidentally breathing a toxic substance. For example, when we smell chlorine gas from a bottle of common household bleach, our reaction is immediate and violent as our eyes water, noses run, and bronchial tubes go into spasm, making breathing difficult. This experiment can be duplicated over and over if we want proof that bleach is directly responsible for a given set of reactions. Of course, most of us learn very quickly that it is the bleach that caused our discomfort, and we decide to be more careful in the future.

In this case, the cause of the discomfort (the bleach) was very closely associated with the effect: the burning eyes, runny nose, and restricted breathing. A simple and very scientific deduction, though slightly sophomoric in this context, can be drawn from this cause-and-effect relationship.

Similarly, hay fever is generally the result of breathing the spores of pollinating grasses and weeds. It normally occurs when these plants are in bloom in the spring or, in warmer climates, closely following a summer rain and the resultant regrowth of the grasses and weeds on the hillsides. Sinus drainage and restricted breathing are the direct and reproducible results of an allergic reaction to an inhalant. But with NAET evaluation, I have found many people suffer from the symptoms of hay fever from an allergy to sugar or spices. When they get desensitized through NAET, their hay fever like symptoms get better.

A proper diagnosis based on a similar cause-and-effect relationship is much more difficult when the cause is, say, olive pollen encountered early in the day by a sensitive person, and the resultant delayed asthma is similar to that experienced when one breathes in the bleach or the grass and weed spores. In addition, it is much more difficult to make a proper diagnosis when a person's physical responses to a given allergen differ radically from those that would normally be anticipated.

Karl, a man in his early 60's, came to my office, nearly incapacitated by lapses of memory and seizures that resembled some form of epilepsy, Alzheimer's disease or perhaps a mild stroke. He retired two years before in excellent health. According to his wife, he did not suffer from any significant illnesses during his entire life. He was not depressed or lonely after his retirement, rather he enjoyed his retirement. He enjoyed gardening and he found happiness and pride in maintaining a well-kept lawn and a vegetable garden without using pesticides. He always enjoyed home-cooked meals and rarely dined out.

He had been healthy when one day, 14 months before I saw him, she found him sitting on the reclining chair on the porch between one of his breaks from mowing the lawn,

staring at the street, unresponsive to her questions. In about five minutes, he woke up from his trance state and behaved as if nothing had happened. He did not remember anything that happened during the previous several minutes. Since it was not anything serious, she did not tell him about it but observed him closely after that. During the next few days she noticed similar episodes a few more times and told him about it. He did not have any memory of such episodes. Then she brought their physician-son into the picture.

The son immediately came over and took him to different doctors. Karl was examined by various specialists who did a battery of tests, tested his blood by all standard laboratory works, performed MRIs and scans a number of times hoping to find a cause to this sudden, strange problem. His son consulted different experts in fields, determined to find the cause. Karl continued to have short lapses of memory and seizures, would often wander off in total confusion or complete amnesia, sometimes losing track of significant blocks of time. Neurological examinations and a CAT scan showed his brain-wave pattern to be completely normal.

After months of searching for an answer to the cause of Karl's problem, and not finding any relief with the usual treatment for seizures disorders (dilantin, etc.), his desperate son decided to search for answers from an alternative medicine perspective. He read about NAET on our website and immediately made an appointment with me for his father.

With considerable detective work in my office with NMST (Neuro Muscular Sensitivity Testing), the procedure that performs the important NAET detective work, the cause in this case turned out to be the airborne spores of a fern

tree Karl had planted in his backyard fourteen months before. With this new knowledge from NMST, his physician-son and I again evaluated his history. His strange behavior started 14 months before. He was very healthy until then. He had these attacks only during daytime. His hobby was mowing the lawn and caring for the garden in his front and back yards. This retired engineer spent many hours in the back yard cleaning and pulling weeds during the day and took pride in maintaining a good-looking lawn and a vegetable garden. His history pointed one hundred percent towards the cause if one carefully evaluated it – something in the garden was causing his problem.

After successful NAET treatment for the fern, Karl's symptoms subsided. He was able to get off all the symptomatic medications given for his assumed seizures. He lived normally after that.

But now with scientific, investigative and million-dollar, diagnostic equipment, most modern physicians tend to overlook the patient's history as a prime diagnostic tool, even though that's what we were taught in medical schools to look at first.

If NMST were taught in all medical schools (allopathic, chiropractic, acupuncture and naturopathic medical schools, etc.) to all medical students and professionals, more doctors could find clues to their patients' problems faster. If I didn't have NMST as a screening tool, I would have missed the diagnosis too. No one with regular medical school training would associate epileptic seizures with a fern tree in the back yard that is planted 150 feet away from the main house.

Karl's reaction to the inhalant was totally illogical and unanticipated, physiologically. The lack of the usual respiratory distress, when compared to other patients who suffered sensitivities to inhalants, delayed diagnosis and treatment for several months by traditional medical specialists. His standard laboratory tests and scans did not produce any noticeable abnormalities. Without any abnormal findings, traditional neurologists could not decide upon a diagnosis or treatment plan. His unusual neurological symptoms of memory lapses, frequent seizures eventually occurring at least five or six times daily during the day, and fatigue were not associated or suspected by the new arrival of a fern tree in his garden by his Western-medicine trained physicians. This added to the frustration and potential danger of the patient.

This points out that there is no typical response to allergens in the real world. If we are depending on allergies to produce a given set of responses for all people, we may misdiagnose and provide wrong treatments. We must remember that since we cannot duplicate and package a cause-and-effect responsive medication as antidote to handle all cases of poisoning from inhaling fern tree spores, or any other allergen, medical specialists must not oversimplify treatment of patients who do not exhibit typical allergic symptoms, whatever we perceive them to be. Otherwise, we risk missing myriad potential reactions that may be produced in some people but not in others in response to contacts with substances that are, for some, allergens.

HAY FEVER

The term "hay fever" describes the symptoms of allergic rhinitis when it occurs in the late summer due to an individual's reaction to ragweeds, sage weeds, fresh flowers and grasses. Hay-fever symptoms result from the inflammation of the tissues that line the inside of the nose (mucus lining or membranes) after allergens are inhaled. Adjacent areas, such as the ears, sinuses, and throat can also be involved.

Hay fever is characterized by symptoms of watery discharge from the nose, eyes, and throat, sometimes stuffy nose, sneezing, post nasal drip (throat clearing), nasal itching (rubbing), itchy ears and throat, loss of taste and smell, and other symptoms similar to those accompanying colds. Many patients also complain of an annoying tickle inside the nose that results in violent sneezing. Others have dry, hacking coughs, and some have a profuse watery secretion of the nasal passages. Allergens, the substances that are foreign to the body, can cause an allergic reaction that results in hay fever symptoms. The three most common symptoms characteristic of hay-fever are severe sneezing, watery nasal discharge, and stuffy nose.

Often, hay-fever victims also suffer from nasal polyps, which are swellings or growths of the mucus membrane that occur within the nostrils. Nasal polyps are caused by congestion and inflammation of the mucous membrane and tend to grow or shrink in accordance with the severity of the symptoms. In some instances, they become large enough to completely block the nasal passages and even extend beyond the nostrils.

NAET evaluation may reveal energy interference in the lung, stomach, spleen, or large intestine meridians. Hay fever can be eliminated in most cases, when the allergens are identified, and desensitized through NAET.

Hay Fever and Bronchitis

I suffered from hay fever and bronchitis since the age of twelve, ever since I moved to Norwalk, California. Dr. Devi treated me for my allergy to yeast, pollens, grasses,

My Pink Eyes

I woke up in the morning with red, watery, itchy, swollen, sticky right eye. I had thick, white, discharge coming out of the right eye. Left eye was slightly pink, no swelling, with minimal watering and discharge. I am a second year medical student, preparing to take a series of exams in the next few days having to take the first one on the same evening. I was afraid that my eye inflammation might continue through my exams and I wouldn't be able to study or take any of them. My mother called an ophthalmologist for an appointment and got one for the next day. But he prescribed me some eye drops. I used it all morning. My pain and symptoms persisted. That is when my mother called Dr. Devi's office for NAET. I got the appointment right away. After examining my eyes, Dr. Devi said I was having a reaction to milk and asked my mother to go home and get a sample of milk I drank previous night before bedtime. As soon as the milk arrived, she desensitized for the milk through NAET. She had to repeat the NAET every fifteen minutes for three times on me. I was in her office for an hour. My eyes were completely normal when I left her office after an hour. I directly went to school and never missed any of my exams. Thank you Dr. Devi, for discovering this amazing technique!

Sam Martin

Buena Park, CA

flowers, perfumes and mold. I have been totally symptom-free for the past 17 years (since 1986).

JannaGossen

La Mirada, CA

ALLERGIC CONJUNCTIVITIS

Allergic conjunctivitis is an inflammatory process involving the tissue layer that covers the surface of the eyeball and inner surface of the eyelids. It is characterized by watery, itchy, reddened eyes (due to vascular dilation), sticky eyelids (due to increased secretion-usually white, ropy, viscous discharge), and swollen eyelids (due to cellular infiltration). It can be acute or chronic. In acute cases, the inflammation occurs as a result of an acute allergic reaction to pollens, fumes or chemicals in the foods, or drinks: sudden onset, initially unilateral, with the inflammation of second eye within one week. The whole process may last about four weeks to completely heal.

In chronic conjunctivitis, repeated exposure to some allergens may be the cause.

Allergic conjunctivitis (acute or chronic) may be caused from environmental allergens like pollens from grass, flower, trees, weeds; foods and condiments; smell from cooking or smoke from barbecuing; chemicals and cosmetics; chlorine, pool chemicals, and products from animals and insects.

NAET evaluation may reveal energy interference in the lung, liver and spleen meridians. Allergic conjuctivitis can be eliminated in most cases, when the allergens are identified, and desensitized through NAET.

Seasonal Allergies

Many individuals suffer from seasonal allergies, allergies to tree pollens, in the northern New Mexico. All of my patients have found relief and improved health through NAET. I am very happy to inform you that many of my patients have eliminated their chronic asthma and allergies permanently. NAET is great!

Denise Aughtman, D.O.M.
1911 5th St., Suite 207
Santa Fe, New Mexico 87505
(505) 670-9455

ALLERGIC RHINITIS

Allergic rhinitis is a very common medical problem affecting more than 15 percent of the population, both adults and children. Allergic rhinitis takes two different forms, seasonal and perennial. Symptoms of seasonal allergic rhinitis occur in spring, summer and/or early fall and are usually caused by allergic sensitivity to pollens from trees, grasses, weeds or to airborne mold spores. Other people experience symptoms year-round– perennial allergic rhinitis. Although allergic rhinitis (inflammation of the nose and nasal passages) causes symptoms similar to hay-fever, the symptoms often persist throughout the year, and are caused by sensitivity to house dust, mites, animal dander, mold spores, inhalants, fabrics, chemicals in the fabrics, or other substances. Many patients suffer from both hay-fever and rhinitis simultaneously, with symptoms considerably aggravated during the pollen season.

Often, patients with allergic rhinitis have no noticeable symptoms of asthma. However, when they are exposed to cold air, exercise or infection they show significant bronchial hyper-responsiveness or asthma-like symptoms. Our first exposure to an allergen is often through the nose or mouth. This exposure can cause coughing, watery eyes, wheezing, hives and even gastrointestinal symptoms.

The principal symptom in children is blocked nasal passages. Children suffering from hay fever or allergic rhinitis tend to breathe through their mouths and have a nasal twang to their voices. If the condition continues untreated, facial deformity frequently results. In addition to the above symptoms, many patients complain of intense itching of the eyes, ears, throat, soft palate and sometimes, the face. With hay fever, the symptoms may vary considerably between patients. Many hay fever patients are very sensitive to changes in temperature and weather. Their condition is usually aggravated by cool or damp air, even though the pollen count is lower under these conditions.

Most sufferers of allergic rhinitis feel better in warm, sunny weather because cold, damp weather patterns frequently cause the patient to feel chills. As a result, asthma patients require more bedding and warmer clothing than most.

Many patients with pollen allergies will also be allergic to certain foods, as well as to other inhalants and contactants. Other than pollens and grasses, the most common items found to cause hay fever are: sugar, carob, corn, wheat, beans, pineapple, tomato, banana, perfume, furniture, cats, dogs, feathers, kapok, dust, plastics, rubber and leather.

NAET Works, Here is the Proof!

J.S. was a four year old boy who had suffered from a total body rash his entire life. He was very ill as an infant and in fact suffered from extreme allergies from the first day of life. At approximately two weeks of age he lost all of his skin in a massive shedding whereupon he was transferred to a university center where he battled for his life for several weeks.

When I first met the boy he had thick scales all over his body, many of which were red and angry looking. His mother was keeping him away from milk and eggs at that time as he had been R.A.S.T. tested. His problem at presentation were his marked eczema with scratching and sores which kept him from sleeping well, inability to go outside because of urticaria and chronic abdominal pains and diarrhea. He was so allergic to egg that even holding an unbroken egg would cause him to break out in hives (this was described as happening many times so I take it at face value).

He underwent NAET treatments going through the major foods and finally chemicals, pesticides and pollens. An interesting feature of his case is that he had IgE levels quantified before treatment and afterwards.

Allergens	Pre-treatment	Post-treatment
Egg white	iv	1
Milk	iv	0
Casein	iv	0
Total IgE	32	9.2

Today J.S. is a very happy boy. He can play outside anytime, eat what he wants and sleeps through the night without itching or needing special creams.

David M. Schultz, M.D.
Leipsic, OH
(419) 943-2130

It is extremely important that hay-fever and rhinitis sufferers consult an appropriate allergist knowledgeable in NAET when their symptoms begin. These conditions have a tendency to become increasingly severe with each season. The possibility of serious complications increases with each severe attack. Untreated patients are also likely to accumulate new allergens, as well as encounter increased sensitivity.

Allergic rhinitis may be also caused by other substances including house dust, chemical sprays, household cleaning chemicals (in housemaids, chemical factory workers, people from janitorial services), occupational dusts (such as flour in the bakery, silica, cement and metallic dusts, industrial dust), chalk powder, marker-inks, coloring crayons (in school children, school teachers, classrooms), newspaper, copying paper, recycled paper, newspaper- ink (writers, people in the newspaper and printing industry), house- paint, water and oil-based paints, plastics, crude oil, formaldehyde, cosmetic agents, soaps, perfumes and other chemical agents.

Prompt treatment of these allergies greatly decreases the likelihood that a comparatively mild allergic manifestation, such as hay-fever or allergic rhinitis, will develop into a more severe allergy, such as asthma.

NAET evaluation may reveal energy interference in the lung, stomach, spleen and large intestine meridians. Allergic rhinitis can be eliminated in most cases, when the allergens are identified, and desensitized through NAET.

ASTHMA

Asthma occurs much more frequently in families that have a history of various allergic conditions. The tendency toward this particular allergic ailment seems to be more frequently inherited than in most other allergic diseases. A woman who suffers from hay fever may have children who suffer from some other manifestations, such as dermatitis, arthritis, (rather than hay-fever). On the other hand, a patient who suffers from asthma is quite likely to have children who also suffer from asthma.

Various allergens from everyday life can trigger asthma in sensitive people.

The Common Triggers Of Asthma

- Food, drinks, vitamins, and drugs
- Environmental allergens: house dust, dust mites, industrial dust, mold, pollen, grass, weeds, animal dander, animal epithelial, etc.
- Air pollutants: cigarette smoke, auto exhaust, smog, chemi cals, perfumes, pesticides, infections in the respiratory tract, etc.
- Weather changes: cold, heat, humidity, fog, dampness, damp-heat and damp-cold
- Exercise: running, aerobics, etc.
- Emotional factors: fear, grief, anger, etc.
- Biohazard agents: industrial waste, insecticides, pesticides.
- Bed material: mattress, pillow, linen, pillow case, etc.
- Building materials: paint, paint thinner, insulation, dry wall, formaldehyde, ceramic tiles, etc.
- Cosmetics: body lotion, makeup, lipstick, hair products.
- Drinks: water, alcohol, soft drinks, coffee, tea, etc.
- Dust: house dust, industrial dust, etc.

- Fabrics: polyester and other petrochemicals-based fabrics, but also nylon, cotton, silk, rayon, etc.
- Flowers, perfume from flowers, etc.
- Food: regular and genetically engineered vegetables, legumes, and fruits.
- Food additives: sulfites, nitrates, M.S.G., food colorings.
- Gasoline and other crude oil products.
- Insect parts and venom: bee, scorpion, mosquito, ant, cockroach, wasp.
- Herbs and herb products: tea, supplements.
- Latex: rubber, elastics, rubber backing or sole of the shoe.
- Lead: lead piping, lead pencils, paint.
- Medications: prescription or over-the-counter.
- Mercury: dental amalgam, fish, pesticides, antibacterial agents.
- Microorganisms: bacteria, viruses, parasites.
- Mold: yeast, fungus.
- Nutritional Supplements: vitamins, minerals.
- Other environmental Substances.
- Paper products: newspaper, toilet paper, books, etc.
- Perfume, cologne, after-shave lotion, soap.
- Plastics: computer keyboard, mouse, household products.
- School work materials.
- Footwear: shoes, socks, slippers.

- Tools: working materials.
- Vinyl.
- Weather conditions like cold, heat, humidity, wind.
- Wood: Furniture, cabinet, tables.
- Cooking smells, smells from coffee brewing, popcorn popping, perfumes, cosmetics, smoke from cigarettes and cigars, wood burning from fireplace, from barbecue, wildfire burning, chemical fumes (smells from paint, washing soaps, detergents, dry cleaning chemicals, household cleaning chemicals, swimming pool chemicals), can also trigger asthma in some people.

Allergens, like pollens, flowers, molds and dusts are the most prevalent cause of asthmatic attacks. In addition, asthma can be caused by allergies to almost any food (fish, shellfish, peanuts, food additives, food colors, sulfites), clothing, chemicals (fabric softeners, detergents, shampoo, body lotion), perfumes, synthetic substances (formaldehyde, plastics, latex, rubber goods, ceramics, tiles, cookware) and natural substances (cotton, leather). Cold, heat, dampness and moisture can cause an asthmatic reaction as well as an allergy to one's spouse, children or another human associate, even, a pet.

Like other allergic conditions, asthma responds very well to NAET. When beginning treatment, it is always better to combine Western medical treatments with NAET for better and faster results. After you are treated for the Basic items, you can request your pulmonologist to evaluate your symptoms and try to gradually reduce the dosage of any medication that you may be taking.

If you suffer from asthma, you should receive prompt allergy treatment. Asthmatics should always carry inhalant sprays for quick relief in emergencies because an asthma attack can unexpectedly be triggered at any time from a contact with any allergen.

Environmental allergens like pollens, grasses, cigarette smoke, cooking gas smell, frying food smell, perfumes, flowers, spices, burning smell, food seasoning smell, chemical smells, smell from fabrics, dust, mold, smell from animals, smell of body secretions (stool, urine, semen, vaginal discharge, sputum, sweat, bad breath), etc., can trigger respiratory discomforts like cough, asthma, post-nasal drip, throat irritation, etc. If you are sensitive to any of the above items that smell, collect them and treat with NAET. The allergen or its smell should not bother you afterwards.

Many people are allergic to the medication they take for relief. When they do not receive the expected relief from their medication, they complain to their doctors. Doctors will change to a different medication and if that doesn't work, move on to another. The doctor's and the patient's frustration can be reduced by learning NMST (Neuromuscular sensitivity testing) techniques to detect allergies and sensitivities. (Read Chapter 6 for details on NMST). Doctors could check the medication using NMST before prescribing it. Pharmacists could check the allergy before they supply the medication to the patient. It is very essential to all practicing medical professionals and pharmacists to learn NMST. You, as a patient, should learn the testing techniques in order to test yourself for the medications you are taking. You can screen allergy to the medications before you take them. This way, you can eliminate the frustration of seeking different doctors and different remedies and still not finding relief.

People with asthma will often have energy interference in the following meridians: lung, large intestine, stomach, spleen, kidney, urinary bladder, liver, gallbladder meridians.

We Enjoy Our Christmas Tree!

My wife's irritating, impossible Christmas tree allergy was eliminated by NAET 9 years ago. Ever since, she is 100 percent free of her Christmas-time Hayfever. We are so grateful to NAET for giving us the freedom to enjoy our Christmas and cherish a fresh tree each year.

Stanley Inouye, D.D.S., M.S.D.
Sacramento, California

EXERCISE-INDUCED ASTHMA

This is a common form of asthma that occurs only when a person exercises. People with chronic asthma can develop symptoms whenever they are exposed to a "trigger" of the asthma, such as a virus, pollen, dust, cigarette smoke or exercise.

About 80 to 90 percent of people who have chronic asthma have exercise-induced asthma. And about 35 to 40 percent of people with seasonal allergies also have exercise-induced asthma. Symptoms worsen during the spring and fall. Exercise-induced asthma tends to particularly affect children and young adults (because of their high level of physical activity) but can occur at any age.

Exercise-induced asthma is initiated by the process of respiratory heat exchange (the fall in airway temperature during rapid breathing followed by rapid reheating with lowered ventilation). The more heat transferred, the cooler the airways become, the more rapidly they rewarm, the more the bronchi are narrowed.

In some cases, cold dry air is believed to trigger exercise-induced asthma. Exercising outdoors in the winter or even mouth breathing can set off the asthma attack. (Breathing through the nose normally warms the air.) Some doctors recommend indoor swimming as an ideal form of exercise because the warm, humid air keeps the airways from drying and cooling.

Exercise-induced asthma is monitored using a peak-flow meter. This hand-held device measures air flow (how fast air is blown out of the lungs). Patients can regularly use peak-flow meters to measure their own air flow. This allows patients to obtain a much earlier indication of an oncoming attack.

In many instances, unpleasant memory-associations from the past regarding exercise can bring on an attack of exercise-induced asthma. In these cases, the emotional issue needs to be sorted out and treated with NAET to prevent further occurrences of this problem.

Pollen Allergy

I have treated many cases of Pollen allergies (Kafun Shou) and environmental allergies successfully with NAET. The following year, none of them had any problems with pollens in our heavy pollen season.

NAET Sp: Teruaki Nozawa, D.C.
2-4 Mitojima-honcho
Fuji-city, Shizuoka,
Japan 416-0924

Traditionally, exercise-induced asthma is managed by avoiding the offending allergic triggers and using medications up to an hour before exercising. Medications help to relax the muscle spasm of the airways, permitting improved air flow. Certain medications can be used to prevent the lining of the airways from swelling in response to cold air or allergic triggers. Inhaled cortisone-related medications are sometimes used to reduce inflammation and swelling in the airways. If you are allergic to cortisone or other medications, you can eliminate that allergy by being treated by an NAET specialist near you.

Many people suffer from exercise-induced asthma. Children, when they take part in sports activities, can get asthma but the exercise itself might not be the direct cause. Some start wheezing when they run on the grass. Sometimes pesticides sprayed on the grass may be the cause. Allergy to fabrics (socks, shoes, shorts, shirts, detergent used in cleaning clothes, etc. can trigger asthma). Sometimes the food they ate before they began exercising can also cause an asthmatic attack. Smell of flowers, smell of freshly cut grass, allergy to grass itself, can cause asthma.

Apart from allergy to external sources, some people react to their internal secretions. During exercise, endorphins and enkephalins are naturally produced. In some people these hormones are not produced or produced only in small amounts during a normal day. But when they exercise, they are generated in larger amounts. If the person is allergic to these endogenous hormones, he/she does not feel good after exercise. In some people the overproduction of these hormones causes adverse reactions like weight gain after regular exercises, feeling depressed after playing tennis, getting angry after running track, etc.

NAET evaluation often will reveal energy interference in the kidney, lung and urinary bladder meridians in people who suffer from exercise-induced asthma.

Sinusitis

Inflammation or infection of any of the four groups of sinus cavities in the skull is called sinusitis. These cavities are opened to the nasal passages. The cavities, located within the skull or bones of the head surrounding the nose, include the:

- Frontal sinuses over the eyes in the brow area,
- Maxillary sinuses inside each cheekbone,
- Ethmoid sinuses just behind the bridge of the nose and between the eyes,
- Sphenoid sinuses behind the ethmoids in the upper region of the nose and behind the eyes.

Each sinus has an opening into the nose for the free exchange of air and mucus, and each is joined with the nasal passages by a continuous mucous membrane lining, therefore, anything that causes a swelling in the nose — an infection, an allergic reaction, or an immune reaction — also can affect the sinuses. Air trapped within a blocked sinus, along with pus or other secretions, may cause pressure on the sinus wall. The result is the sometime intense pain of a sinus attack. Similarly, when air is prevented from entering a paranasal sinus by a swollen membrane at the opening, this can also cause pain. Sinusitis is not the same as rhinitis, although the two may be associated and their symptoms may be similar. The terms "sinus trouble" or "sinus congestion" are sometimes wrongly used to mean congestion of the nasal passages. Most cases of nasal congestion are not associated with sinusitis.

The location of your sinus pain depends on which sinus is affected. Headache when you wake up in the morning is typical of a sinus problem.

Pain over the frontal sinuses is felt when touched on the forehead; infection in the maxillary sinuses can cause your upper jaw and teeth to ache and your cheeks to become tender to the touch; inflammation of the ethmoid sinuses cause swelling of the eyelids, tissue around eyes, pain between the eyes, tenderness on the sides of your nose, loss of smell, and a stuffy nose, because they are located near the tear ducts in the corner of the eyes. Sphenoid sinuses are less frequently affected; infection in this area can cause earaches, neck pain, and deep aching at the top of your head. Other commonly seen symptoms are fever, fatigue, cough, runny nose or nasal congestion.

Most people with sinusitis, however, have pain or tenderness in several locations, and their symptoms usually do not clearly indicate which sinuses are inflamed.

From the NAET standpoint, an allergy to environmental agents, foods, chemicals, household cleaning chemicals, fabric softeners, newspaper ink, formaldehyde, chlorine gas, water-filter chemicals, bleaching agents, etc., can cause energy disturbance in the stomach and large intestine meridians and can cause sinusitis. If sinusitis is allowed to continue, it can eventually turn into asthma.

BRONCHIOLITIS

This is an inflammation of the bronchioles or small passages in the lungs. Children under age two are especially vulnerable. This infection can be caused by several kinds of viruses. Allergy to foods, and chemicals in foods (like food additives and colorings in soft drinks, candies, etc.) also can mimic bronchiolitis. Symptoms can include a runny nose, slight fever, coughing, and wheezing. NMST can help identify the source of the causative agent. If the cause is found, treatment can be easy. One must either avoid the allergen or get treated by NAET.

BRONCHITIS

Bronchitis is characterized by an infection of the bronchial tree with resultant bronchial edema and mucus formation. Because of these changes, patients develop a productive cough and signs of bronchial obstruction, such as wheezing or shortness of breath on exertion. The inflammation in acute bronchitis is transient and usually resolves soon after the infection clears. In some patients, however, the inflammation can last several months. In rare cases, a postbronchitis cough can persist for up to six months.

Bronchitis can have causes other than infection. Bronchial wall inflammation can occur in asthma or can be secondary to toxic exposure such as smoke from cigarette, or a chemical fume inhalation in chemical factory workers. It is important to realize that when underlying inflammation is present, such as in asthmatics or smokers, infectious agents are likely to cause more severe cough and wheezing.

Viruses are the most common cause of bronchial inflammation in otherwise healthy adults with acute bronchitis. Nonviral agents cause bronchitis in a small percentage of people. Only a small portion of acute bronchitis infections are caused by nonviral agents like Mycoplasma pneumoniae and Chlamydia pneumoniae. The major portion of bronchitis is started from exposures to various allergens: food additives, food preservatives, contaminated foods, chemical fumes, swimming pool chemicals, chemicals in the fabrics, contaminated bottled drinking water, city water, pesticides, etc. Water chemicals in the city water are changed periodically in certain cities in the USA. In the first few weeks after the change of chemicals, many sensitive people seem to get an epidemic of upper respiratory infections, eventually leading to bronchitis. During these weeks, hospital emergency rooms and doctors' offices are overflowing with victims of upper respiratory tract infections and bronchitis. Once we recognized the pattern of this yearly or twice a year epidemic, we began educating our patients to boil and cool the water before consumption. This alone reduced the infection by huge percentages among our patients and their families. Some people can be still sensitive to the chemicals even after boiling. In those cases we treated them for the chemicals with NAET.

According to one of the reports released by CDC, in the United States alone, the evaluation and treatment of bronchitis is estimated to cost $200 million to $300 million per year, not to

> An 11-year old girl had severe sinusitis for two years. Her family had a water filter that had been installed two years previously. She was treated with NAET for the water chemicals and her problem was eliminated. Now, one year after treatment, the family is still using the same filter system without any trace of prior symptoms.

mention the cost of losing time at work, missing other activities and suffering the physical discomfort.

CHRONIC BRONCHITIS

Repeated irritation to the respiratory system is the cause of chronic bronchitis. It may be from virus, bacteria, allergic agents like cigarette smoke or chemicals. If acute bronchitis is not taken care of, it can eventually become chronic. The major symptom is the irritable, frequent cough. Cough becomes more frequent during the daytime and even at night, disturbing sleep. The patient then notices that activities previously tolerated well, now cause shortness of breath and perhaps some wheezing. As the disease progresses, shortness of breath may be caused by very ordinary activities such as getting dressed in the morning or having a bath. The patient with advanced bronchitis may be unable to walk or climb stairs without supplemental oxygen. He or she may be confined to a chair or bed because of shortness of breath and the type of heart failure which may develop in the late stages of this disease. Minor chest infections in patients with severe chronic bronchitis may require intensive treatment in the hospital. As the disease can wear on and on and the sufferer becomes more and more debilitated, it becomes an important cause of disability.The annual cost of this disease in terms of time lost from work, disability pensions and medical therapy may approach many millions.

From the NAET standpoint, if any illness does not respond to traditional treatment (antibiotics, herbals, etc.), continues to remain as chronic, the irritant is constantly accompanying the person everywhere- that means the person is not free from the irritating substance even for a minute. NAET specialists look for the cause in the daily consumed food, drinking or bathing water, chemicals, fabric detergent, softener, or other allergens that can be causative factors leading to chronic bronchitis.

A 34-year-old female suffered from chronic bronchitis for over a year. When she came to me for evaluation, she had gone through many courses of antibiotics, was on oxygen support, and leading a miserable life. In this case,

NMST detected fabric softener as the causative agent. She had changed the fabric softener just over an year before and continued to use that one ever since. When we identified the source, I encouraged her to stop using all fabric softeners for awhile instead of treating the fabric softener with NAET. We wanted to see how soon she became free of symptoms when avoiding the allergen. To remove softener residue, we asked her to double rinse all the fabrics in the house including her clothes, wash cloths, bath towels, bed linen, sofa cover, etc. She was also asked to air out her house by opening windows and doors letting the air take away the smell left from the fabric softener. She moved out of the house for a few days. After a week, when she returned to the office for treatment, her bronchitis was almost gone. Then she was desensitized for the fabric softener with NAET. After that she was free from her bronchitis. Even though the allergy was gone, she was too fearful to use the same fabric softener again. She said, "The painful memories of the past year were enough to last a lifetime!"

EMPHYSEMA

This is a disease of the alveoli that results in shortness of breath. Allergy to smoke, inhaling toxic fumes for a prolonged period (fire smoke, cigarette smoke, toxic fumes, pesticides, etc) can cause this. Chronic bronchitis and asthma, if left untreated, can turn into emphysema. This is a disease in which there is destruction of the walls of the air sacs of the lung, and it is frequently preceded by chronic bronchitis. Emphysema adds to the breathlessness suffered by the patient with chronic bronchitis.

PNEUMONIA

This is an inflammation of the lungs, usually caused by infection. In my experience, the primary cause or trigger may be an allergy (an allergy to milk, juice, sugar, etc.), then as a second step, the infection begins. A milder form of pneumonia is called "walking pneumonia." A doctor may use this term to describe pneumonia that isn't severe enough to cause bed rest.

According to one report, every year, more than 60,000 Americans die of pneumonia — an inflammation and infection of the lungs. Although pneumonia is a special concern for older adults and those with chronic illnesses, it can strike young, healthy people as well.

There are more than 50 kinds of pneumonia that range in seriousness from mild to life-threatening. In infectious pneumonia, bacteria, viruses, fungi or other organisms attack your lungs, leading to inflammation that makes it hard to breathe. Pneumonia can affect one or both lungs. Infection of both lungs is sometimes popularly referred to as double pneumonia.

In many cases, pneumonia follows a common cold or the flu, but it also can be associated with other illnesses or occur on its own. It's best to do everything you can to prevent pneumonia, but if you do get sick, recognizing and treating the disease early offers the best chance for a full recovery. Make sure to contact your NAET Specialist as well as the pulmonologist.

Allergies can lead to pneumonia. Just like any other infections, if you lower your immune system by overexposure to various allergens, opportunistic infectious agents can find their ways into your body and continue to affect you as long as the immunity remains low.

COUGH VARIANT ASTHMA

Cough is the main noticeable symptom among little children. They may be normal during the day. But, in some cases, when they go to bed they begin coughing. Eventually their coughing will end up in wheezing and shortness of breath.

In these children, the major culprit may be traced to something in the bed. Bedroom materials can cause cough variant asthma not only in children but in adults. The common allergens causing cough and asthma at night, can be in the mattress, pillow, pillow case, stuffed toys, plastic toys, plastic sheets, crib toys, reading books, remote control for the TV, pajama, other night-wear clothes, socks, toothbrush, tooth paste, mouth wash, tap water, the night air, night blooming plants if the window is left open, house plants in the bed room, bed room furniture, curtains, drapes, carpets, ceramic tiles, bathroom slippers, depending on what kind of materials one has in the bedroom.

Many people love eating chocolate and enjoy drinking coffee and other caffeinated drinks. Many people are allergic to chocolate and coffee and, in them, allergy to these items can cause asthma.

COOKWARE INDUCED ASTHMA

Asthma, cough, and respiratory disorders can be caused by cooking pans, Teflon coating on the pans, cooking sprays, etc. in sensitive people. The kitchen utensils, silverware and cutleries, other cleaning materials like scrubbers, dishwashing soap, and aroma and smells from: cooking, frying and seasoning, burnt food, popcorn popping, coffee brewing, meat cooking, old kitchen trash, spoiled food, rancid oils, smell from unclean garbage disposal, cleaning chemicals, etc., can produce respiratory symptoms (asthma, sinusitis, coughing spells, dusty feeling in the throat, hay fever-like symptoms and sensation of choking) in sensitive individuals.

SMOKE INDUCED ASTHMA

The smell of cigarette smoke can trigger asthma in sensitive individuals. Such people have to isolate in their own house most of the time. They cannot go out in crowds, or in shopping malls, entertainment parks, restaurants or bars, etc., for fear of asthmatic attacks. Lately, smoking is restricted in many areas of the country. Even so, smokers find their way to pollute public areas with smoke, making it hard for smoke-sensitive individuals to live a normal life. NAET can eliminate the allergy to smoke.

If you are sensitive to smoke, you might also be sensitive to other fumes in the air. Fireplace smoke, smoke from wild fires, smell from coffee brewing, popcorn popping, cooking smell, smell from gasoline, automobile exhaust, etc., can also trigger asthma.

It is helpful to use air purifiers in the house if you are sensitive to these smells. There are many chemical and odor-free products available to help alleviate your symptoms. During the initial NAET treatments, such aids will be beneficial.

ALLERGY TO BODY FLUIDS

I have treated many men and women who developed asthma after they got married. The culprits were traced to the partner's clothes, perfume, hair sprays, aftershave lotion, body odor, etc. We had several women allergic to their husband's semen, urine and saliva. Some suffered from severe yeast-like infections, itch-

From My Satisfied Patients

NAET has transformed the treatment of asthma in many of my cases. It's a great reward to hear a patient say: "I don't really understand these NAET treatments, but they work. I can breathe again without the help of medication. I don't get any more asthma attacks. Even though I carry the asthma medication with me, I rarely need to take them. I can eat many things now and I can go to many places that were forbidden for me before. Thank you, for giving me a new lease on my life!"

I thank you, "Dr. Devi," for bringing this remarkable addition into the armamentarium of the healing arts.

Peter R. Holyk, M.D., F.A.C.S.,
Sebastian, FL (561) 388-5554

ing and dry coughs that did not respond to any medication. When they were treated for these fluids, their problems cleared up.

ASTHMA IN PREGNANCY

Pregnant women with asthma should avoid asthma triggers, including specific allergens such as house dust mites and animal dander, and irritants such as cigarette smoke until they get treated with NAET. If a pregnant woman gets treated for all known allergens during pregnancy, she may not have to take much asthma medications during pregnancy or gestation. In addition, it has been seen that going through all classic NAET treatments (described in Chapter 8) during pregnancy can assist in having a healthy baby.

Household Chemical Triggered asthma

Marina, 28, cleaned houses for a living. She had suffered from severe asthma ever since she began working. She was on three different medications to keep her asthma under control. Often she had to go to the emergency room when her asthma got severe. One of her friends gave her a copy of the Spanish edition of the book, "Say Good-bye to Illness." She immediately decided to try NAET. After she was treated for the NAET basics, she was treated for chemical mix and two other combinations: chemicals with D.N.A, and Chemical mix with heat. Soon after these treatments, her asthma got better.

Mala Moosad, R.N., L.Ac., N.D., Ph.D.
Buena Park, CA

CHILDHOOD ASTHMA

The most common serious chronic disease of childhood, affecting nearly five million children in the United States is asthma. The most prevalent symptoms in children are: coughing, chest tightness, shortness of breath and wheezing. Asthma is the cause of almost three million physician visits and 200,000 hospitalizations each year. In infants and children, asthma may appear as cough, rapid or noisy breathing in and out, or chest congestion, without the other symptoms seen in adults.

If the child has a family history of asthma and allergies, he/she should be tested with NMST for all known or suspected allergens in the child's environment including everyday foods and drinks.

Asthma symptoms can interfere with many school and extracurricular activities. Parents may notice their child has less stamina during play than his or her peers, or they may notice the child trying to limit or avoid physical activities to prevent coughing or wheezing. Normal breathing should be quiet; a child with asthma has noisy breathing.

Often, recurrent coughing spells may be the only observable symptom in young children. Up to 80% of children with asthma

Free From Life-threatening Asthma!

Since I have started treating patients with NAET, the results have been phenomenal, greater than my wildest expectations. Children who had life threatening asthma are now symptom-free. Young adults who were unable to go to university, school, or even walk down the street because they were hypersensitive to the environment, can now go to nightclubs without ill effect. My practice has expanded by at least 200% since treating patients with NAET. Thank you, Devi, for coming to Australia and imparting this wonderful technique which has enabled me to bring health to my patients.

NAET Sp: Maria Colosimo N.D.
Melbourne, Australia

develop symptoms before age five. Some children may wheeze from respiratory infections, which will be relieved when the infections go away. Persistence of wheezing may indicate asthma, which should be treated as soon as possible with NAET to avoid future complications and long-term effects.

Children should be checked and treated for allergens like dust mite, cockroach droppings, animal dander, animal epithelial, pollens and molds. Children are very sensitive to molds. Please make sure there are no molds growing in your bathrooms, under the wash basin, under the shower faucet, swimming pool, old abandoned jacuzzi near bedroom, etc. Children are also very sensitive to cigarette smoke. Please make sure no one smokes around your children.

Cosmetics Triggered Asthma

A teacher became asthmatic when a particular teacher's aide was sent to assist her with activities. The aide was wearing a particular perfume to which the teacher was found to be very allergic. After treating for the perfume, she didn't suffer from asthma when the particular teacher's aide came to assist her.

ASTHMA FROM OCCUPATIONAL HAZARDS

Asthma can be produced by various household chemicals, cleaning chemicals, tanning or cosmetic chemicals, and the chemicals in the work area. Sometimes asthma may be manifested from one's own life-style, living habits, or as offshoots of inherited allergies from parents or grandparents. Various chemical agents around us are capable of producing asthma in sensitive individuals. It is better to check all the possibilities of genetically transmitted allergenic offshoots in certain cases of asthma, emphysema or chronic respiratory problems when they do not respond to medication or other treatments.

Many people are allergic to underarm deodorants and antiperspirants, causing skin rashes, irritation of the skin, dermatitis, boils, infections, lymph gland swelling and pain. The chemicals in the antiperspirants and deodorants are toxic and carcinogenic to some people. Many of these products do their intended job, that is to prevent sweating, by blocking the sweat glands. That could lead to inflammation of the sweat glands, and constant irritation and inflammation can lead to more chronic disorders. After successful desensitization of these products through NAET, the adverse effects of these products can be reduced or stopped.

My Asthma Patients Are Happy

NAET is truly the medicine of the future. It is exciting to be using it in the present. The results and satisfaction are mind boggling. I can hardly believe it, even though I see the results over and over again, each and every day. The scope of the many health problems especially people with asthma is astounding. All my asthma patients can breathe again with the help of NAET. The only problem is there are not enough hours now to treat the many patients wanting treatment with this wonderful technique.

NAET Sp: Terry Power
BSc., Grad DC, M. ChiroSc, D. Ac.
Port Macquarie
NSW, Australia

3

Categories of Allergens
Part-2

As mentioned in Chapter 1, asthma and many other illnesses are caused by disruption of the brain's "Software" program. As such, asthma is an allergic condition in which your lungs and respiratory tract have become sensitive to your environment. An allergen is a substance that induces an allergic reaction. An allergen can be one of the causes of asthma. Once causes are determined and treated by NAET, asthma can often be permanently eradicated.

Common allergens are generally classified into nine basic categories based primarily on the method in which they are contacted, rather than the symptoms they produce.

1. Inhalants (See Chapter 2)
2. Ingestants
3. Contactants
4. Injectants
5. Infectants
6. Physical Agents
7. Genetic Factors
8. Molds And Fungi
9. Emotional Stressors

Ingestants

Ingestants are allergens that are contacted in the normal course of eating a meal or that enter the system in other ways through the mouth and find their way into the gastrointestinal tract. These include: foods, drinks, condiments, drugs, beverages, chewing gums, vitamin supplements, etc. All of these are potential allergens that can trigger asthma in sensitive individuals. In addition, we must not ignore the potential reactions to things that may be touched and inadvertently transmitted into the mouth by our hands.

An estimated 40 to 50 million Americans have allergies. But according to statistics released, only one to two percent of all adults are allergic to foods or food additives. Eight percent of children under age six have adverse reactions to ingested foods; only two to five percent have confirmed food allergies. Allergic reactions to foods typically begin within minutes to a few hours after eating the offending food. The frequency and severity of symptoms vary widely from one person to another. Mildly allergic persons may only suffer a runny nose with sneezing, while highly allergic persons may experience severe and life-threatening reactions, such as asthma or swelling of the tongue, lips or throat.

The most common symptoms of food allergy involve the skin and intestines. Skin rashes include hives and eczema. Intestinal symptoms typically include vomiting, nausea, stomach cramps, indigestion and diarrhea. Other symptoms can be asthma, with cough or wheezing; rhinitis, often including itchy, stuffy, runny nose and sneezing; and rarely, anaphylaxis, a severe allergic reaction that may be life threatening.

In the individual with food allergy, the immune system produces increased amounts of immunoglobulin E antibody, or IgE. When these antibodies battle with food allergens, histamine and other chemicals are released as part of the body's immune reaction to these substances. These chemicals can cause blood vessels to widen, smooth muscles to contract and affected skin areas to become red, itchy and swollen. These IgE antibodies can be found in different body tissues - skin, intestines, and lungs - where specific allergy symptoms such as hives, vomiting, diarrhea and wheezing are observed.

Although food allergy occurs most often in infants and children, it can appear at any age and can be caused by foods that had been previously consumed without any problems. Finally, excessive exposure to a particular food may affect the overall rate of allergy to that food, as testified to by the high prevalence of fish allergy among Scandinavians and of rice allergy among the Japanese. Eggs, cows milk, peanuts, soy, wheat, tree nuts, fish and shellfish are the most common foods causing allergic reactions, but almost any food has the potential to trigger an allergy. Foods most likely to cause anaphylaxis are peanuts, tree nuts and shellfish.

Keep in mind that if you are allergic to a particular food, you might be allergic to related foods. For example, a person allergic to walnuts may also be allergic to pecans and persons allergic to shrimp may not tolerate crab and lobster. Likewise, a person allergic to peanuts may not tolerate one or two other members of the legume family such as soy, peas or certain beans. Some people know exactly what food causes their allergic symptoms. They eat peanuts or a peanut-containing product and immediately break out with hives. Other individuals need their allergist's help in determining the "culprit", especially when the specific food cannot be identified or when the symptoms show up many hours after ingesting an offending food.

According to CDC, more than 95 million Americans are affected by some type of digestive condition. Specifically, over 60 million people experience heartburn at least once a month, 20 million suffer from ulcers at some point in life, and 138,000 new cases of colorectal cancer are diagnosed each year.

Although anyone can develop a food allergy, there is a hereditary component. Children with one allergic parent have about twice the risk of developing a food allergy than children without allergic parents. If both parents are allergic, a child is about four times more likely to develop a food allergy than if neither parent is allergic.

Many children with food allergies also show sensitivity to inhaled allergens such as dust, cat dander and pollen, or may develop allergies later in life. In addition, adults who develop food allergies often have histories of respiratory allergies such as asthma.

The most common symptoms involve the gastrointestinal tract, beginning with swelling or itching of the lips, mouth and/or throat. Once the food enters the stomach, nausea, vomiting, diarrhea or cramping may occur. Itching, hives and skin rash or redness also are common. Severe cases can result in anaphylactic shock — extreme difficulty in breathing, irregular heart beats, fainting, etc. and if not treated immediately, it can be fatal.

Allergic reactions to food usually begin within minutes to hours after eating the offending food. In a very sensitive person, simply touching or smelling the offending food may produce an allergic reaction. Even being kissed by someone who has eaten peanuts, for example, can cause a reaction in severely allergic individuals. Anaphylaxis is a rare but potentially fatal condition in which several different parts of the body experience allergic food reactions at the same time. Symptoms may progress rapidly and include severe itching, hives, sweating, swelling of the throat, breathing difficulties, lowered blood pressure, unconsciousness or even death. If you are experiencing such a reaction, seek emergency medical care immediately!

People think the terms food allergy and food intolerance mean the same thing; however, they do not. A food intolerance is an adverse food-induced reaction that does not involve the immune system. Lactose intolerance is one example of a food intolerance. A person with lactose intolerance lacks an enzyme that is needed to digest milk sugar. When the person eats milk products, symptoms such as gas, bloating, and abdominal pain may occur.

According to the information from traditional allergy associations (American Academy of Allergy, Asthma & Immunology, Food Allergy Network), currently, there are no medications that cure food allergies in traditional medicine. Strict avoidance is the only way to prevent a reaction. They believe most people outgrow their food allergies, although peanuts, nuts, fish, and shellfish are often considered lifelong allergies. But according to them, there is definitely no cure. But through NAET, many thousands with such severe food allergies have received lifelong relief from their symptoms.

Epinephrine, also called adrenaline, is the medication of choice for controlling an anaphylactic reaction. It is available by prescription as an EpiPen® auto injection. People with such severe allergies should carry this with them all the time.

Other food allergy-related health disorders like Crohn's disease, irritable bowel syndrome, leaky gut syndrome, acid reflux disorders (heartburn), gastric ulcers, diarrhea, constipation, vomiting, respond well to NAET.

HEARTBURN/GERD

Heartburn, also called acid indigestion, is a burning pain in the chest that occurs when stomach acids flow backward into the esophagus. Sixty million Americans experience heartburn at least once a month and more than 15 million have heartburn symptoms daily. Persistent heartburn that occurs two or more days a week is often a sign of the more serious disorder known as gastroesophageal reflux disease (GERD), or acid reflux. Many people with gastroesophageal disease also suffer from cough and asthma. In many cases, heartburn can be controlled with over-the-counter medicines and life-style modifications, such as quitting smoking, losing excess weight, not eating close to bedtime and avoiding certain foods. If acid indigestion persists despite these changes, it could be gastroesophageal reflux disease (GERD), a serious form of heartburn. When GERD is left untreated, complications can occur, including severe chest pain or bleeding of the esophagus. GERD responds well to NAET treatments. Find a nearest NAET practitioner and start the treatments right away. When GERD is under control, asthma gets better too.

PEPTIC ULCER

A peptic ulcer is a sore on the lining of the stomach or the beginning of the small intestine. The most common symptom is a burning pain in the stomach. The bacterium Helicobacter pylori is now recognized as the cause of almost all cases of peptic ulcer disease. Traditional treatment generally involves antibiotics given with acid suppressing other medications. Due to various reasons, the acid production in the stomach gets disrupted and causes various digestive disorders. This also triggers asthma in some people. One of the causes for disrupted acid production is allergy to foods and often one's own stomach acid itself. Find your allergies using the instructions in Chapter 6, and find a practitioner near you to get a series of NAET treatments to correct the problem.

ALLERGY TO NUTRIENTS

Some people are found to be allergic to nutrients in the food they have consumed on a daily basis since infancy. These nutrients, vitamin C, B vitamins, minerals, vitamin A, etc., are essential for maintaining normal health by assisting the body to prevent toxic buildup and to help repair usual wear and tear. Nutritional allergies cause asthma in some people. When people are allergic to the essential nutrients, they do not respond to usual asthma therapies or medications.

FOOD ADDITIVES CAUSED ASTHMA

It is very hard to find pre-made foods without food additives and preservatives. They are necessary to maintain the appearance, shelf-life, texture and taste. They cause various health problems including asthma and other respiratory disorders in sensitive people. M.S.G. (monosodium glutamate or accent) and Sulfites are widely publicized substances that have been added as a preservative to salads and potatoes in restaurant salad bars and in the fast food industry. The intention was to maintain freshness (or at least the appearance of freshness, flavor and shelf-life) as these vegetables sit out in display cases for long periods of time. Unfortunately, sulfites are salt derivatives of sulfuric acid, to which many asthma sufferers are highly allergic.

The area of ingested allergens is one of the hardest to diagnose, because the allergic responses can be often delayed from several minutes to several days, making the direct association between cause and effect very difficult. This is not to say that an immediate response is not possible. Some people can react violently in seconds after they consume the allergens. In extreme cases, one has to only touch or come near the allergen to signal the central nervous system that it is about to be poisoned, resulting in symptoms that are peculiar to that particular patient. Usually, more violent reactions are observed in ingested allergens than in other forms.

Literally any substance we eat can become an allergen for someone who is sensitive to any ingredient in the product. For instance, people have been known to faint every time they eat an orange, without exhibiting any other food allergies. By avoiding this allergen they can prevent the occurrence of an allergic reaction and may find it unnecessary to subject themselves to regular medical care. However, one should keep in mind that in this and similar minor allergy cases, patients who are not treated tend to manifest allergic symptoms to other similar allergens in the future. For example, a patient who fainted when she ate a banana might develop asthma or migraine headaches when she eats an orange at a later date. She may be allergic to potassium, one of the basic ingredients in the banana and orange.

We live in a highly technological age. New substances are being introduced into our diets that preserve color, flavor and extend the shelf life of our foods. Some additives used in foods as preservatives have caused severe health problems. Some artificial sweeteners cause mysterious problems in some people and may mimic various serious diseases, such as asthma, skin problems, arthritis, toothache, multiple sclerosis, acute prostatitis, trigeminal neuralgia, vertigo, chronic dry cough, joint pains and sciatica, to name a few. Most of these additives are harmless to most people but can be fatal to some who react to them.

Cheese causes asthma and respiratory problems in many people. Tyramin, a protein found in cheese, especially in aged cheese, is found to be one of the culprits for triggering sinusitis and asthma in some people. Yeast as in bread can cause cough and asthma in sensitive people.

FOOD COLORING

Food coloring causes many allergies. Young school-going children consume various food colorings in large quantity in various forms: ice cream, candies, chewing gums, etc. Many children suffer from asthma, sinusitis, cough, hyperactivity, poor concentration, irritability, autistic behaviors, hives, rashes, itching, eczema, etc. These common symptoms can be expected of food colorings, when ingested by sensitive people. Unusual symptoms like adrenal depletion, profuse sweating after eating food colorings confuse the patients and the physicians.

WATER CHEMICALS

City water and bottled spring water cause misery to asthmatic populations. Chemicals added to tap water changes very often. You need to regularly test your tap water and drinking water for a possible allergy to the newly-added water chemicals in order to prevent surprises.

ALLERGY TO MILK AND MILK PRODUCTS

Milk proteins are known to cause asthma, sinusitis, and other upper respiratory problems in sensitive people. Homogenized milk causes concern to a lot of asthmatic patients in the United States. Even after they clear for the milk allergy through NAET, homogenized milk drinkers can face allergic reactions once in awhile. This depends mainly on cattle feed. It was found out from various dairies that they have no control over what the cows are fed daily. Most of the nut-oil companies, after extracting the oils, dry the leftovers into compact cakes and sell them to the dairies. In the dairies, these cakes are randomly fed to the cows. When the cows secrete milk, some of the substances from the nuts are also secreted through the milk. Sometimes, if the cows are fed with hay and grasses that are sprayed with pesticides, these substances are also excreted in the milk. When an allergic person drinks this milk, he/she can react at any time. This particular reaction is not due to any allergy to milk but to the pesticides or other ingredients in the milk. This should be kept in mind when treating for a milk allergy.

ALLERGY TO MEDICATIONS

Medications are clearly beneficial. However, some medications may cause adverse physical, physiological and emotional reactions in some people. Many asthmatics react to their asthma medications. The very drug that is supposed to help you breathe better often makes them have more shortness of breath, insomnia, dry mouth, dry throat, cough, joint pains, ankle swelling, indigestion, gastrointestinal symptoms, mainly diarrhea, heart palpitation, nervousness, skin rashes, itching, etc. Many people complain that the antibiotic erythromycin causes gastrointestinal symptoms such as diarrhea. Chemotherapeutics cause nausea, vomiting, hair loss, skin problems, and brown spots on the skin surface. These types of reactions are due to an allergy to the drug, which means that the patient's immune system is overreacting to the drug but may not be high enough to produce measurable antibodies. If there is no adverse reaction, drugs can do their expected job.

These reactions may be IgE mediated or non-IgE mediated. IgE mediated reactions are known to be true allergic reactions. Non-IgE mediated reactions are known as simple hypersensitivity reactions. Most standard laboratory tests are not able to record hypersensitivity reactions because the immune system is not involved in the initial stages. That means doctors have no definite means of demonstrating your mild to moderate allergic sensitivity to the drugs through laboratory works. Muscle Response Testing described in Chapter 6 is the only source of dependable testing available now to detect your sensitivities. Whether they are mild or severe, NMST can detect it. Check your allergy to the drugs you are taking using this method before you take them. If you find an allergy, please find an NAET practitioner near you and treat your allergy. You will be surprised to enjoy the magical benefits of the drugs on your asthma if you are not adversely reacting to them.

Symptoms of sensitivity reactions can vary and they can be triggered by any drug. Some people may be able to take the drugs in lower doses and get some benefit even though they may be bothered by some mild sensitivities. Some drugs interact with each other and cause undesired reactions or severe adverse reactions if taken together. Some asthma drugs and antibiotics should not be mixed together. Please consult with your doctor or pharmacist. Sometimes if prescribed blindly, one may receive more of the drugs than required. That can also cause reaction in the body. Overdosing should be avoided. It can be toxic and trigger symptoms, especially if given for a long period of time. Some drugs may interact with certain foods or cause abdominal bloating or flatulence. The combination of food and drug may be inhibiting the function of digestive enzymes. Taking extra enzymes may be helpful at times. All these mild to severe reactions can be tested through NMST and NAET treatments for food combining, food and drug combining, or drug combining can solve such abdominal discomforts.

Some people with asthma or sinus problem, have a sensitivity to aspirin and other non-steroidal anti-inflammatory drugs. Up to 19% of adult patients with asthma, and up to 40% of those with nasal polyps (growths) or chronic sinusitis, experience aspirin sensitivity. This sensitivity may not be an IgE mediated reaction, but often symptoms can be severe. Those with aspirin or NSAID sensitivity may experience symptoms such as nasal congestion and a runny nose; itchy, watery or swollen eyes; cough; difficulty breathing or wheezing; or hives on the skin. In rare instances, these types of severe reactions can result in anaphylactic shock. If your symptoms are severe, seek emergency medical help immediately. If you are seeing a NAET practitioner, you should tell him/her about your sensitivity to aspirin, so that he/she can treat you appropriately.

Great care must be taken while testing and treating for these types of drugs or foods because it might help to get a better prognosis when you know what other ingredients are in the products. If everyone could get proficient in muscle-response testing, most hazardous accidents from food and drug allergies could be prevented by testing before consuming any foods or medications.

Contactants

Contactants produce their effect by direct contact with your skin. They include the well-known poison oak, poison ivy, poison sumac, cats, dogs, rabbits, cosmetics, soaps, skin cremes, detergents, rubbing alcohol, gloves, hair dyes, various types of plant oils, chemicals such as gasoline, dyes, acrylic nails, nail polish, fabrics, formaldehyde, furniture, cabinets, etc. Most contactants are also included in the environmentals and they all are known to produce asthmatic symptoms in sensitive people.

Allergic reactions to contactants can be different in each person, and may include asthma, eczema, skin rashes, hives, sinusitis, cough, etc. It is apparent that something contacted by the skin can produce symptoms as devastating to the patient as anything ingested or inhaled.

NAET is Very Effective in Treating Asthma!

As a neurologist, I have seen many diseases as a direct result of allergies. I knew of no other better way of locating the causes of asthma and treating them successfully, which is natural, safe, noninvasive and drug-free. NAET treats most common and uncommon allergies in the most efficient way in few minutes.

Ravinder Singh, M.D.
Beverly Hills, California
(310) 278-4171

Woolen clothes may also cause asthma and allergies in people. We have seen people who cannot wear wool without breaking out in rashes. Some people who are sensitive to wool also react to creams with lanolin base, since lanolin is derived from sheep wool. Some people can be allergic to cotton socks, orlon socks, or woolen socks with symptoms of knee pain, etc. People can also be allergic to carpets and drapes that could cause knee pains and joint pains.

We had a few other female patients who were allergic to their panty hose and suffered from asthma, leg cramps, high blood pressure, swollen legs, psoriasis, and persistent yeast infections. Toilet paper and paper towels also cause problems to asthmatics.

Food items, normally classified as ingestants, may also act as contactants on persons who handle them constantly over time. Cooks who knead wheat flour daily could suffer from respiratory disorders like asthma, emphysema or even angina or coronary heart diseases. People who cut vegetables and pack them in the grocery stores could suffer from asthma and sinusitis or any other respiratory disorders. They may be allergic to the vitamin C from the vegetables. Some people suffer from asthma by continuous exposure to certain vegetables and food products like cutting and canning peppers or onions.

Other career-produced asthma and allergies have been diagnosed for cooks, waiters, grocery-store keepers, clerks, gardeners, etc. Virtually no trade or skill is exempt from contracting allergens.

Injectants

Allergens are injected into the skin, muscles, joints and blood vessels in the form of various serums, antitoxins, vaccines and drugs. As in any other allergic reaction, the injection of a sensitive drug into the system runs the risk of producing dangerous allergic reactions. To the sensitive person, the drug actively becomes a poison, with the same effect as an injection of arsenic. No one would intentionally give an injection of a potentially dangerous drug to a person. However, some drugs seem to become more allergenic for certain people over time, without the person being aware of the potential risk. Take the increasing incidents of allergies to the drug penicillin as an example. The reactions vary in people, from hives to asthma to anaphylactic shock and death.

Most of us do not often consider an insect bite in the same way as we would an injection received from a physician or a member of his staff, but the result is quite the same. At the point of the bite, a minute amount of the body fluid (saliva) of the insect is injected into the body. These fluids may be incidental to the bite. They may be simply secretions normal to the salivary gland or biting part of the insect, or they may be a necessary part of the biting mechanism, such as the saliva of the mosquito, which is formulated to keep the host's blood from coagulating so blood extraction is not difficult. These fluids may also be specifically formulated to produce immobilizing pain, in order to protect the insect from its own predators, such as the spider that uses its bite to secure food and inflict pain in the defense of its territory, the bee that uses its sting for defense, and the wasp that uses its sting to obtain food and defend its nest.

Certain animal bites also inject near-lethal amounts of toxins into the bloodstream of victims, again to immobilize the prey and to protect itself from its own predators, and other animals.

Bites from mammals also fit into this category. They include children's bites which can produce considerable infection at the site of the bite, and the injection of the dreaded virus from the bite of an infected animal.

The normal reaction to a bite, other than that to the obvious lethal bites, ranges from mild swelling around the site of the injection, a mild reddening and, of course, a slight to moderate discomfort in the body from attempting to free the toxin that produces itching. Rarely are these bites and stings lethal to the normally insensitive person.

For some people, however, a sting or a bite by an animal or insect is potentially lethal. Even a single mosquito bite may produce an extreme and sudden onset of edema (the abnormal collection of fluids in the body tissue and cells) and severe respiratory distress. There have been many cases of anaphylactic shock, respiratory and/or cardiac failure in sensitive persons, following the slightest insect bite.

Infectants

Infectants are allergens that produce their effect by causing a sensitivity to an infectious agent, such as bacteria. For example, when tuberculin bacteria is introduced as part of a diagnostic test to determine a patient's sensitivity and/or reaction to that particular agent, an allergic reaction may result. This may occur during skin patch, or scratch tests done in the normal course of allergy testing in traditional Western medical circles.

Infectants differ from injectants as allergens because of the nature of the allergenic substances; that is, the substance is a known injectant and is limited in the amount administered to the patient. A slight prick of the skin introduces the toxin through the epidermis and a pox or similar harmless skin lesion will erupt if the patient is allergic or reactive to that substance. For most people, the pox soon dries up and forms a scab which eventually drops off without much discomfort. However, for those individuals who are reactive to these tests, it is not uncommon to experience fainting, nausea, fever, swelling (not only at the scratch site but over the whole body), respiratory distress, etc.

In other words, the introduction of an allergen into the reactive person's system runs the potential risk of causing a severe reaction, regardless of the reason or the amount of the toxic substance used. Great care must be taken in the administration of tests that are designed to produce an allergic reaction.

Various vaccinations and immunizations may also produce such allergic reactions. Some children after they receive their usual immunization get very sick physically and emotionally.

It should be noted that bacteria, virus, etc. are contacted in numerous ways. Our casual contact with objects and people exposes us daily to dangerous contaminants and possible illnesses. When our autoimmune systems are functioning properly, we pass off the illness without notice. When our systems are not working at maximum performance levels, we experience infections, fevers, etc.

From a strictly allergenic standpoint, however, contact with an injectant does not produce the expected reaction for that particular injectant; rather a more typical allergic reaction takes place, as can be seen in the tuberculin test as an example. It is clear that the reaction to the test would probably not be a case of tuberculosis but rather a mild allergic response such as an infectious eruption under the skin.

Physical Agents

Heat, cold, sunlight, dampness, drafts or mechanical irritants may also cause allergic reactions and are known as physical allergens. When the patient suffers from more than one allergy, physical agents can affect the patient greatly. If the patient has already eaten some allergic food item, then walks in cold air or drafts, he/she might develop upper respiratory problems, sore throat, asthma or joint pains, etc., depending on his/her tendency toward health problems. Some people are very sensitive to cold or heat, whether they have eaten any allergic food or not. Such cases are common.

Many asthma patients have exaggerated symptoms on cold, cloudy or rainy days. These types of patients could suffer from severe allergy to electrolytes, cold, or a combination of both.

Some patients react violently to weather changes, getting asthma during a cloudy day, not responding to their medication. These patients have hypo-functioning immune systems due to poor absorption of nutrients, especially trace minerals. When they finish the treatment program, they do not continue to get asthma with weather changes.

Genetic Causes

Discovery of possible tendencies toward allergies carried over from parents and grandparents opens a large door to achieving optimum health. Most people inherit the allergic tendency from their parents or grandparents. Allergies can also skip generations and be manifested very differently in children.

Many people with various allergic manifestations respond well to the treatment of various disease agents that have been transmitted from parents.

Parents with rheumatic fever may transmit the disease to their offspring, but in the children the rheumatic fever agent may not be manifested in its original form.

Molds and Fungi

Molds and fungi are in a category by themselves because of the numerous ways they are contacted as allergens in everyday life. They can be ingested, inhaled, touched or even, as in the case of Penicillin, injected. They come in the form of airborne spores, making up a large part of the dust we breathe or pick up in our vacuum cleaners; fluids such as our drinking water; as dark fungal growth in the corners of damp rooms; as athlete's foot; and in the particularly obnoxious vaginal conditions commonly called "yeast infections." They grow on trees and in the damp soil. They are a source of food, as in truffles and mushrooms; of diseases such as ring worm and the aforementioned yeast infections, and of healing, as in the tremendous benefits mankind has derived from the drug Penicillin. These items cause asthma, sinusitis, bronchitis, cough in many people.

Reactions to these substances are as varied as other kinds of allergies. This is because they are a part of one of the largest known classifications of biological entities. Because of the number of ways they can be introduced into the human anatomy, the number of reactions are multiplied considerably. Fungi are parasites that grow on living as well as on decaying organic matter. That means that some forms are found growing in the human anatomy.

One reacts to one's own body secretions like urine, stool, sweat, etc. Fungus or mold can grow anywhere in the body, where the area is fairly moist and not exposed to sunlight or air.

They are contracted by contact and is often passed from person to person anywhere there is the potential for contact (i.e.gymnasiums, showers, locker rooms and other areas where people share facilities).

No More Anaphylaxis to Bee Stings!

My son, Evan, who, three years ago had an anaphylactic shock when he was stung by a bee, was stung again by a bee about two weeks ago. I have treated him with NAET for anaphylaxis to bee stings since the original sting. His reaction to the recent bee sting was a red wheel at the site of the sting. But he did not need the anaphylaxis treatment and he is doing fine.

Thank you, Dr. Devi, Mala, Mohan for teaching me this fabulous NAET treatment technique, so that I could cure my child from his severe anaphylactic reaction to bee stings, that is not treated successfully to full recovery by any other medical disciplines.

NAET Sp: Anthony DeSiena, D.C.
Eugene, Oregon 97401,
(541) 686-BACK (2225)

Allergies to cotton, orlon, nylon, or paper could result in the explosions of infections including Ascomycetes fungi (yeast) that women are finding so troublesome. Feminine tampons, toilet papers, douches, and deodorants can also cause yeast infections and asthma.

Emotional Stressors

Many times, the origin of physical symptoms can be traced back to some unresolved emotional trauma. Each cell in the body has the capability to respond physically, physiologically and emotionally to our daily activities. When the vital energy flows evenly and uninterrupted through the energy pathways (acupuncture meridians), the body functions normally. When there is a disruption in the energy flow through the meridians (an increase or decrease), energy blockages can occur, causing various emotional symptoms in those particular meridians. According to Oriental medical theory, there are seven major emotions that can cause pathological health problems in people: sadness affects lung meridian, joy affects the heart, disgust affects the stomach, anger affects the liver, worry affects the spleen, fear affects the kidney, and depression affects the pericardium meridian. Please read Chapter 7 for more information.

Emotional factors can trigger cough, asthma, sinusitis, bronchitis or any other upper respiratory disorder. Emotional upsets, such as death, divorce, problem at work, or in the family, even unresolved arguments can produce respiratory problems like cough, sinusitis, asthma, shortness of breath, blocked nostrils, and various other physical or physiologic symptoms.

During NAET evaluation, the NAET doctor—before proceeding with the treatments—checks out all these factors. If practiced regularly, it takes only awhile to rule out unusual factors. A NAET practitioner is well-trained to test and determine emotional influences.

A Few Case Studies and Testimonials

A teenager had appetite only for pasta and tomato sauce every day. He lived on that. He refused to eat any other food. He suffered from asthma. He was receiving allergy shots from an allergist. He was introduced to NAET by his sister who had great results with NAET for her fibromyalgia symptoms. In the office, I detected vitamin C was again the culprit. But this time tomatoes were the main vitamin C ingredient he consumed. After he was treated for vitamin C and the spaghetti sauce, his asthmatic symptoms reduced greatly.

A 32-year-old woman suffered from asthma every night after retiring to bed. She was reacting to the toothpaste and tap water that she used every night at bedtime. After she was treated for toothpaste and water, she was freed from her asthma.

A nurse, 43, came in with a strange problem. During the day she suffered from cough and asthma. In spite of her asthma medication, she continued to cough and wheeze through the day. She worked day shift, which started from 7a.m. and ended at 7 p.m. As soon as she reached home, she removed her work clothes and settled into comfortable home clothes. She attributed her cough and asthma to the various smells in the hospital where she worked. I treated her for the NAET Basics; she felt better overall. But her asthma did not reduce. After the Basics, she was evaluated again and I detected that she was reacting to the synthetic bras she wore. On questioning her, she told me that she never wore a bra at home. She put it on only when she went to work or went to visit friends or family. After she was treated for her bra, she stopped having asthma.

John Ray suffered from severe asthmatic attacks in the middle of the night. When he came to the office he was found to be allergic to many items. After completing the Basics he was reevaluated since his asthma was not getting better. He was found to be allergic to the wood frame of his bed. After he was treated for the wood, he felt better and eventually got complete freedom from his asthma.

A 44-year-old woman had a history of asthma since childhood. Finally, through NAET, the cause was traced to her allergy to bamboo. The bamboo caused an energy blockage in her lung meridian. It was discovered that both her childhood home and current house were decorated with bamboo and cane furniture. Her asthma improved when she completed the treatment for bamboo.

A 36-year-old female suffered from asthma ever since she began working as a secretary in a law office. The reason for her asthma was traced to the nylons she was wearing to work daily. When she was treated for nylons her asthma got better.

John Rick was one week old when his mother found him one day in his crib without any signs of life. He wasn't breathing. She grabbed him and shook him. Her husband called the paramedics. Within three minutes, paramedics arrived and found his heart had stopped. They used a defibrillator and revived him. John was alive once again, his breathing and heartbeat restored. He was taken to the hospital for monitoring for 48 hours, after which he was sent home with a beeping monitor. Whenever he stopped breathing, the beeper went off. Back home his beeper was going off frequently, at least five to eight times a day. His mother, grandmother and father watched closely for 24 hours

around the clock. Although he was doing fine at the hospital, he was having breathing stoppages frequently at home. Later on, it was found that he was allergic to the fancy, attractive, plastic crib covering and other plastic accessories. After he was treated for these plastic items by NAET, he did not have the problems again.

Margaret, 78, suffered from asthma for the past four years. She never had asthma before. NAET testing detected that her nightgowns were the causative agents. She was treated for the clothes and her asthma got better instantly.

A 40-year-old male baker at a pizza place suffered from severe asthmatic attacks almost daily. He was allergic to the wheat flour that he used in making the dough. After he was treated for the wheat, his asthma symptoms reduced.

Mary, a piano teacher with acute asthma, complained of wheezing every time she played the piano. It was discovered she was allergic to the ivory of the keyboard.

Sam, a school teacher, complained of cough, chest tightness, and shortness of breath every time he traveled in his car. He was allergic to the leather seats. After he was treated for the leather he didn't complain anymore.

A ten-year-old boy began wheezing by the time he reached the classroom in the morning. He was allergic to his school bag.

Another, a 12-year-old boy had asthma daily at 10 a.m around morning break, only on school days. He was found to be allergic to the carrots and celery he brought for snack to the school every day.

Another, a 13-year-old suffered from asthmatic attacks daily in his math class. He was found to be allergic to the math textbook.

Helene, 74, liked to drink cold water, but she always choked on icy cold water. She also developed an allergic dry cough whenever she ate ice cream. She was treated for all the ingredients in the ice cream, yet her coughing spells and choking incidents persisted. She was finally treated for actual ice cubes. Afterwards, she could enjoy ice water and ice cream without choking.

A four-year-old boy suffered from asthma in the Winter. During the summer he was OK. He was allergic to the cold. After treating for cold, and cold-damp, his asthma said good-bye to him. Last year his parents took him to the ski mountain. They reported later that he did very well during the two night's stay at the mountain cabin. He didn't have any asthma.

A 34-year-old male suffered from mild to moderate wheezing in the shower. He tried to take a quick shower everyday. If he stayed a few minutes extra in the shower, his asthma got worse. Then he had to go for a convention to be held in Kauai. As he came out of the airplane he felt his chest tightening and before he knew it, he was having an asthmatic attack right in the baggage claim area. He used the ventolyn spray. It usually helped him. But this time it did not help. He was standing just outside the men's toilet near the water fountain facing the wall, arms rested on the wall, head resting on his bent elbow, struggling to breathe. One of the NAET practitioners who was going to the female toilet spotted him struggling to breathe. She immediately sensed the cause of his asthma to be the heat and high

humidity in the air. She went to the bathroom looking for a container to get hot water. There was an empty can of cottage cheese in the trash bin. She took the container and rinsed it with water, filled it with hot water from the bathroom and came to the man who was struggling to breathe.

She held the container with hot water to his face and advised him to breathe the mild humid vapor in the air and at the same time dip his fingers in the hot water. The water was just hot. Not enough to produce vapor. But having him feel the water by his fingers and smell the humidity outside, she fooled his brain by simulating NAET treatment for humidity. She continued to give him NAET treatment in that standing position. By the time she finished the NAET treatment on his back, his breathing became better. Later she found out that he was an NAET practitioner himself and they were both going to attend the same NAET convention at the Kauai-Sheraton which I was conducting. Once in the hotel, she repeated the NAET for humidity every two hours for three more times that day. The next morning he said he never felt better. He did not have any more asthma through the NAET convention nor during the stay in Hawaii.

Monica, 48, suffered from severe asthma for four years. She had been on hormone supplements for the four years. She was found to be allergic to provera, the hormone supplement. After she was cleared for provera her asthma symptoms relieved.

A 17-year-old female student suffered from asthma since infancy. She was on a number of sprays and medications including cortisone. Nothing seemed to give her the needed relief. She was evaluated in our office. Her parents did not

suffer from asthma but her grandfather did. She was found to be allergic to many common allergens. She immediately began with our NAET program. When she finished the NAET Basics, she felt better overall. Her energy improved but she continued to get asthma daily. She was reevaluated and found to be reacting to tuberculosis bacilli itself. Her grandfather had died from tuberculosis. She carried his genes. She was treated for the energy of tuberculosis and for the first time in years got relief from her asthma.

A woman who suffered from bronchial asthma was cleared of her asthma when she was treated for the energy of pneumococcus, the bacterium responsible for pneumonia. Both of her parents had died of pneumonia soon after her birth.

Ray, a man of 44, responded well to the treatment for the energy of diphtheria, thus clearing his chronic bronchitis. He had inherited the tendency toward allergies from his mother, who almost died from diphtheria when she was seven. The reaction to diphtheria was manifested in him as bronchitis, sinusitis and arthritis.

Jill, 55, suffered from shortness of breath due to the Epstein-Barr virus and various allergies. After treatment for the energy of the virus, her response was very encouraging. Upon questioning her, it was found that her Japanese parents, uncles and aunts died of tuberculosis. She was immediately tested and treated for the energy of tuberculosis and she became allergy free and healthy once again.

Sara, 42, had severe migraines all her life. Her mother had rheumatic fever as a child. Treatment for rheumatic fever lessened her migraines. She was free of her migraines when she completed NAET basic 15 and a few from the NAET Classic allergen list (Read Chapter 8). She hasn't had another migraine since 1991.

But one of her female children suffered from severe asthma since infancy. Prior to NAET treatments, the parents had to take her to emergency room three to four nights a week since she did not respond to the medication they used at home. Her daughter was also treated for all NAET Basics and a few NAET classic allergens. Her asthma condition improved but she continued to suffer from other upper respiratory infections like bronchitis, pneumonia, etc. with exposures to atmospheric changes, cold air, smoke, etc. She was desensitized for all atmospheric allergens: cold, heat, humidity, dampness, etc. Then we treated her for the energy of the bacteria that was responsible for rheumatic fever in her grandmother and she hasn't had another asthma attack or much of upper respiratory infections since 1992. She is a 24-year-old, young woman with a full-time career and lives in San Diego. During the fire disaster of San Diego in October 2003, she lived in the community shelter with the fire smoke everywhere, and helping other victims to survive the tragedy. After everything settled, she called to report that she never had any sign of asthma, or respiratory problems even though she was breathing the charcoal particles and black smoke all day and night while she was at the shelter. Many people at the shelter had to be taken to the hospital due to their asthma and other respiratory problems. She kept her epi-pen on hand but she never had to use it.

A 23-year-old man suffered from repeated bronchitis, cough, and low grade fever for over an year. He took many courses of antibiotics during this time without satisfactory results. While he was on antibiotics, he felt better. Soon after he stopped them (after the completion of the prescribed course), within the next couple of days, his bronchitis and upper respiratory problems returned. Then he was referred to me by his physician for allergy evaluation. Through NAET testing procedures, I found his chronic bronchitis was due to an allergy to mold. When we desensitized for mold, he continued to sleep on his flotation water bed at night and the treatments began failing repeatedly. After failing for fourth time, NAET testing detected that his water bed had some mold in it and that was the cause of the treatment failure. He could not understand how the mold inside the water bed can affect him to cause continuing bronchitis for more than an year. He said his water bed was securely zipped inside another bag, heavily padded with a thick layer of foam), he had added the water treatment remedy to the water. New to NAET procedures, he was still skeptic about NAET testing and treatments. He went home to look inside the water bed to see if there was in fact any mold.

He was surprised at the discovery he made when he looked into the water bed bag. There was a mild leak at the bottom of the water bed and the lower part of the bed was getting wet. The leak was huge enough to wet the foam pad on top. Then he looked inside the water bed to see the quality of the water for any growth and possibly to take a sample of the water to be checked by me next day. The water inside the king size water bed had turned into a black moldy mass. He threw away the bed completely after saving a sample to bring to me next day. After the treatment for that sample, he did not fail again. His yearlong bronchitis said goodbye to him with that treatment and has not returned in three years. He is a firm believer of the validity of NAET testing now.

A five-year-old boy was addicted to bottle-feeding. He felt comfortable with bottles and he refused to eat food any other way. His mother had to puree all his food and feed him through the bottle with a large hole in the nipple. This became his routine. Mother wanted to wean him off the bottle but every time she would take away his bottle and try to spoon-feed him, he would develop flu symptoms and fever ranging from 102-104 degree Fahrenheit. Then he would lose his appetite and refuse to eat any food. The child cried for hours. Crying caused upper respiratory problems, so his worried mother would give him the bottle again. As soon as he had the bottle, his fever would come down to normal and he would fall asleep. When he woke up, he would be normal again.

It was very difficult to break this habit. When the family took him to Hawaii on vacation, they told him that they forgot to bring the bottle with them, but when he got back he could have the bottle again. Until then, he would have to eat like his mom and dad did. He was also bribed with a toy. He agreed to this arrangement. With different activities in Hawaii, he forgot about the bottle for a week. When they returned, he did not like to drink from the bottle anymore. Our brain adapts to new habits easily.

One of my patients, a 54-year-old female lawyer, developed her asthma six years ago on the same evening when she had her root canal work done at the dentist's office. She was allergic to gutta purcha tissue used during root canal work.

Another woman suffered from severe daily asthma that did not respond to medications for seven years. She was allergic to a water filter that was installed seven years ago.

A 60-year-old woman suffered from her nighttime asthma for 20 years after she began sleeping on a water bed 20 years before.

One of my patients reported that her son's asthma began a few days after he received a kitten for his birthday.

Another patient developed asthma after she worked in her garden for three days. She was found to be allergic to the fertilizer. A young boy developed asthma whenever he ate vegetables from his garden even though they were grown without any artificial fertilizers or pesticides. He was found to be allergic to the dirt from his back yard.

A gardener suffered from asthma every time he mowed the lawn, put in a flower bed, or trimmed a tree. He had to give up his job due to uncontrolled asthma. He was simply allergic to the tools of his trade: flowers, grasses, weeds, trees, and pollens. After receiving a series of NAET treatments for the environmental agents he was able to resume his job as a gardener.

A seven-year-old boy developed asthma after he was stung by a bee and was hospitalized for the bee sting for a week. He got over the bee sting reaction, but went home with asthma. He was allergic to the drugs he received in the hospital.

A four-year-old boy was highly allergic to milk, egg, wheat, beef, and nuts. His older brother was not allergic to most foods. The family began cooking and eating the

items that the young boy was not allergic to. The older boy felt deprived of his favorite foods. He began temper tantrums trying to hurt his younger brother when no one was watching him. He felt the younger brother was taking all fun out of his life. Finally, the parents realized their mistake. They found a solution. One of the parents took him to the nearest park, and got his favorite food for him to eat. After eating in the park, he washed his hands and brushed his teeth before he came to the house. This worked. The older boy felt special by this special loving treat by his parents and felt more loving towards the younger brother who was less fortunate than he. The younger boy took about two years to take care of all of his known allergies and now they both can consume anything they want.

Vitamin C Triggered Asthma

A 28-year-old woman had a history of asthma since childhood. She knew that she was allergic to milk and milk products. She avoided them. She continued to get asthmatic attacks every night. Through NAET I detected her to be very allergic to vitamin C. She was reacting to all the vegetables, fruits and other substances that contain vitamin C. She was also taking 2000 milligrams of vitamin C daily to help boost the immune system. She drank orange juice, grapefruit juice and lemonades daily because she craved them. Vitamin C caused her asthma. When she was successfully treated for vitamin C, her asthma stopped.

Allergic to Table Salt

A 48-year-old woman suffered from asthma since childhood. She was found to be allergic to table salt. When she was successfully treated for salt, she found freedom from her asthma.

Allergy to Rice Krispy

Steve, a young man in his early teens, had come to the office for a sports-related injury. He also had a history of asthma. On one occasion, his mother brought to the doctor's attention that he experienced repeated sinus troubles and continuous itching in an area four finger widths below the knee, on the outer side of the anterior tibial crest. The itching was on the stomach meridian, which meant that the cause of the allergic rash was related to something he was eating frequently. On questioning him further, it was revealed that whenever he ate his favorite breakfast cereal he broke out in a rash.

A simple experiment was set up for confirmation of the effect of the cereal. He was given all his breakfast items: juice, toast and rice cereal, one by one. Then he was given time to chew. All went well until he placed one, and only one, rice cereal flake in his mouth and chewed. He immediately complained of feeling hot and began to redden in an allergic rash, and in a few more seconds he had almost slipped into an anaphylactic shock. After several tense minutes and continuous treatment by NAET, his symptoms subsided.

Peanut Allergy of a Little League Player

In a similar, but unfortunately more tragic instance, peanuts were responsible for the death of an otherwise healthy 12-year-old boy in Midwestern United States. Although he knew that he was allergic to peanuts, he acci-

dentally ate them as an ingredient in cookies after a Little League game. He died shortly after reaching the hospital in anaphylactic shock.

My Asthma Medicine Caused My Asthma!

I used to get severe asthmatic attacks. I was told to take asthma medicine. Whenever I took it, my asthma got worse. Dr. Devi discovered that I was allergic to it. She treated me and now I can take my medication to reduce my asthma.

Mary B.

Anaheim, CA

From Permanent Disability to Fully Active Life!

The doctors had told me that I would be permanently disabled and that the medicine I was taking was to the absolute limit. That was when I could not walk across the floor without sitting down and resting because my breath was so short from the asthma I had suffered with for 12 years. A friend had told me about Dr. Devi, but I thought I would wait for awhile because I had no experience with acupuncture. But finally, I decided that I had no choice but to go, see and find out what would happen.

My life has not been the same ever since! Previously, I had been tested for all kinds of allergies and the doctors I had gone to had told me that my asthma was from emotions, not allergies, because the testing I had done did not show anything significant. Devi tested me with the muscle weakness test and that showed I was allergic to almost everything I was coming in contact with, including my medication and my husband.

Since coming to her, I have been able to walk, bicycle, eat foods that I no longer react to because of the treatments. I am a voice teacher and had thought I would not be able to sing any longer. Now I am singing, my medicine dosage is minimal, and I am living a life that I did not think, for me, would ever again be possible.

Thought my life was, for the most part, over—as far as living normal. That is not true, and with Dr. Devi's help, I am living a normal life now.

Margaret Brazil

Fullerton, CA

I am Free From Asthma for 18 years!

I came to Dr. Devi through a friend in 1985. I suffered from asthma since childhood. During the last seven years before I saw Dr. devi I developed severe sinusitis. I was on antibiotics at least 20 days a month. My symptoms were sinus headaches, shortness of breath, coughing, and wheezing. Within the first two months of beginning NAET, my sinus headaches were reduced by 90 percent. By then the coughing and wheezing were virtually gone. I was treated by NAET for 8 months and I was completely free of symptoms. Previously I tested positive for grasses, pollens and trees. As per her advice I waited for 10 months more after completion of NAET to do a traditional allergy testing (RAST). I tested negative for grasses, pollens, and trees this time. I am free of asthma and sinusitis for the past 18 years! Thanks to Dr. Devi and NAET.

Greg A.,

Anaheim, California

Exercise Induced Asthma

A 16-year-old female suffered from exercise-induced asthma for seven years. On examination she was found to be allergic to many of the food groups from NAET Basics. She began treatment. After the egg treatment, she had an emotional response; She began sobbing. I retested the egg; this time she was found to be weak on the emotional level. NAET testing and patient-doctor discussion and detective work can get to the bottom of emotional responses. In this case, her kidney meridian was imbalanced. It was determined that she had an unresolved trauma that happened at age nine in relation to a female, non-family member and the category was fear and running. She couldn't remember anything significant that happened at that age. But later her mother remembered the incident: She was at a picnic in one of the parks in the Los Angeles area. She and two other friends decided to run on the park's running track. She was leading ahead of the two and suddenly met with a group of policemen and other people crowded near a dead body of a female who had been discovered minutes before. This female had been killed by the hillside strangler. She took a quick look at the body; her friends didn't get a chance before the police blocked the area and everybody was asked to leave. After that she began getting asthma upon any type of exertion, like running, fast walking, aerobics, etc. After she was treated for the fear of that incident, her exercise induced asthma never bothered her again.

My Allergy to the Environment

I want to thank Dr. Marcia Costello for introducing me to NAET. It has changed my life in so many ways. As you know, I have suffered from allergies/hay-fever since youth. I have been treated on and off for years. The most significant were shots in the late 70's to mid 80's at which time I was declared, "cured". I still had problems in the spring

and fall, however. In the 90's I turned to over the counter medicines at times double and triple dosages to survive. On March 15, 1994 I started homeopathic cure process which was effective. I have not had medication since. However, I have suffered while mowing grass (headaches and wheezing) and in the spring and fall with flowering trees and falling leaves. This is all history now. I had a lot more problems that were masked by a constant congestion and ill feeling that I just got used to. Another problem I had was my body getting used to any new environment when I traveled. Even with the homeopathic "cure" I would feel like I had a flu for a day when I would go from Boston to Minnesota (my home state) then again for a day going to visit relatives in South Dakota from there. The reverse was also true returning back. So in a one-week vacation I probably felt like my old-self and enjoyed myself for 3-4 days, that is if there was no fresh cut grass. Well, now the rest of the story: You introduced me to NAET. My initial complaints were problems breathing while cutting grass and arthritis. Your first treatment was for chicken and feathers. Two days later I mowed grass and for the first time without a breathing problem and residual headache. What can I say!!! Marvelous! Let's go on: After clearing for calcium my diagnosed (through CT scan) osteoarthritis pain in my clavicle joint started to subside to the point it is essentially gone now. As you know I could hardly get a shirt on because of the restriction and pain. After clearing the sulphur my arthritis is almost gone. After mold treatment, I was more clearheaded and freer of breathing problems. The oak treatment again enhanced clear headedness, more focus and calmer demeanor. The most recent treatment that made the most miraculous change, namely for flowers and perfume two weeks before my mother passed away. When the flowers arrived at the funeral home I thought I would be in serious trouble. To my surprise hardly an effect... no headache or congestion, etc. Later the flowers were brought to the home, which again my body was able to adapt

and have no problems or side effects. Now we have the beautiful flowering trees which in the past ruined my spring. This is the first spring that I have enjoyed walking and enjoying the trees and beauty... no headaches, congestion, etc. I am overjoyed. I just returned from a trip to Minnesota and South Dakota. I enjoyed every day! No getting used to the new environment each part of the trip as in the past. I love to golf in the morning, which in the spring is the worst time because of the pollen and fresh cut grass (golf courses mow the grass early in the morning). I would react to these allergens by developing neck and shoulder tightness and tension, obviously, the worst spot on the body to ruin a golf game. That so far is no longer a problem and my golf game has improved. Finally, I had mucus build up during the night and especially bad upon getting up. That symptom is virtually gone. I can finally wear the teeth night guard that my dentist insists I wear. I could not previously wear it through the night because of my congestion which is now gone and I can now protect my teeth at night by wearing the night guard. I have probably missed some of the other changes and look forward to further improvements. Again thank you for your effective NAET treatments. It has been painless and without the side effects of drugs.

Regards

Dave

NAET practitioner:

Marcia Costello, R.N., M. Ac., L.Ac.

Trinity Building 31 Springhill Ave.

Marlborough, MA 01752

Relief from Constant Colds

I suffered from constant colds and sore throats for over six months. I had taken several courses of antibiotics without getting any relief of my symptoms. I was so desperate and restless. My quality of life went to zero level.

Then one of my friends told me about NAET. All these antibiotics I took all these days never gave me any relief. What can a holistic treatment like NAET do for my incurable disorder? I asked my friend. She replied, "In fact I can't explain to you how NAET works. But it produces magical results!"

When I made my initial appointment, I was told to take a long all the supplements and medicines that I was taking on a daily basis. So, off I went, armed with a box full of vitamins and medicines. The practitioner tested me and told me to stop taking vitamin C pills that I had been taking three times a day for the past six months. She told me that I was very allergic to vitamin C.

I started with the BBF treatment on the first day with some skepticism. The muscle testing and treatments all seemed like a lot of hocus pocus to me. But I responded wonderfully to the very first treatment and felt much better. It seemed that several of my energy pathways were totally out of balance. My practitioner had to balance my body before she treated me each time. Vitamin C was the fifth treatment since my body needed some other treatments first.

I could not believe the difference! My colds and sore throat completely vanished upon passing the treatment for vitamin C. If only I had known about NAET earlier, I would

not have had to endure all the suffering that I did during several months.

Diana Hobson,

Bombay, India

My NAET Sp: Meher Davis, Bombay, India.

4

Detecting Allergies

Symptoms of allergy vary from person to person depending upon the status of the immune system, age of the patient, severity of disease or degree of involvement of the organs and systems, and degree of inheritance. An allergy is a hereditary condition. An allergic predisposition is inherited, but may be manifested differently in family members.

There are many types of conventional allergy tests available to detect allergies; however, if it is done properly, the most reliable and convenient method of allergy testing is NMST (Neuro Muscular Sensitivity Testing). This is a variation of kinesiological muscle testing. Allergies can be tested by NMST and treated effectively with NAET. Please read Chapter 6 for more information on NMST.

Nambudripad's Testing Techniques (NTT)

NTT consists of a number of standard diagnostic tests from Oriental medicine, allopathy, and chiropractic. They are described below:

Tests From Oriental Medicine

1. HISTORY

A complete history of the patient is taken. A symptom survey form is given to the patient to record the level and type of discomfort the person is experiencing.

2. PHYSICAL EXAMINATION

Observation of the appearance, breathing pattern, mental status, face, skin, eyes, color, posture, movements, gait, tongue, scars, wounds, marks, body secretions, etc.

3. VITAL SIGNS

Evaluation of blood pressure, pulse, skin temperature, rate of breathing, and palpable energy blockages as pain, swelling, or discomfort in the course of meridians, etc.

4. NMST

NMST (Neuro Muscular Sensitivity Testing) is the body's communication pathway to the brain. Through NMST, the patient can be tested for various allergens. NMST is based on the principles of *I Ching*, a 6,000 year old Chinese diagnostic modality.

It is closely related to MRT (muscle response testing), a standard test used in Applied Kinesiology to compare the strength of a predetermined test muscle in the presence and absence of a suspected allergen. If the particular muscle (test muscle) weakens in the presence of an item, it signifies that the item is an allergen. If the muscle remains strong, the substance is not an allergen. More explanation on NMST will be given in Chapter 6.

5. DYNAMOMETER TESTING

This is a great tool to test one's own allergy as well as others. Hand-held dynamometer can be used to measure and compare interphalangeal muscle strength (0-100) in the presence and absence of a suspected allergen. The dynamometer is held with thumb and index finger and squeezed to make the reading needle swing between 0-100 scale. Initial base line reading is observed first, then during contact with an allergen. The finger strength is compared in the presence of the allergen. If the second reading is more than the initial reading, there is no allergy. If the second reading is less than the initial reading, then there is an allergy. For example—if the initial (base line) reading without holding an allergen (for example - an apple) is 40 on a scale of 1-100, and if the reading while holding the apple is 28—the person is allergic to the apple. If the second reading is 40 or above, then there is no allergy. Another benefit of dynamometer testing is that the degree of the weakness/strength is measured in numbers and shown on the face. This gives the tester a numeric value about the allergy which is easily understood.

6. ELECTRO-DERMAL TEST-EDT(NAETER)

After the NMST, the Skin Resistance Test (SRT) is administered. The patient is tested on a computerized instrument (Naeter) that is designed to painlessly measure the body's electrical conductivity at specific, electrically-sensitive points (acupuncture points) on the skin, particularly on the hands and feet. The computerized tester also helps determine the various intensities of the allergies based on a 0 - 100 scale. The machine is designed to test food, environmental and chemical allergies, as well as allergies to molds, fungi, pollens, trees, grasses, proteins, vitamins, drugs, radiation, etc. It can be used to test allergies and their intensities before and after treatment so we are able to compare and study the body's response to the treatment.

The procedure does not involve breaking or puncturing the skin. There is no pain or discomfort. Hundreds of allergies can be tested on the patient in minutes. Since the testing probe only touches the skin for less than a second for each allergy tested, this method can be used in testing infants and children as well as adults. Another advantage of this machine is that it has a computer monitor where the patient can read his/her own allergies as they are being recorded. A printout is produced and the data is saved for future comparison.

7. SIT WITH THE ALLERGEN IN YOUR PALM

NAET patients are taught to test the allergen in another easy and safe way. Place a small portion of the suspected allergen in a baby food jar or glass tube and ask the person to hold in her/his palm touching with the fingertips of the same hand for 15 minutes to 30 minutes. An allergic person will begin to feel uneasy when holding the allergen in his/her palm for awhile giving rise to various unpleasant symptoms: begin to get hot, itching, hives, irregularities in heart beats (fast or slow heart beats), nausea, light headedness, shortness of breath, etc. Since the allergen is inside the glass tube, when such uncomfortable sensation is felt, the allergen can be put away immediately and hands washed to remove the energy of the allergen from the fingertips. This should stop the reactions immediately. In this way, the patient can detect the allergens easily.

Traditional Allopathic Testing Procedures

8. SCRATCH TEST

Western medical allergists generally depend on skin testing, (scratch test, patch test, etc.), in which a very small amount of a suspected allergic substance is injected into the person's skin through a scratch on the skin or via injection using a needle. The site of injection is observed for any reaction. If there is any reaction at that area of injection, the person is considered to be allergic to that substance. Each item has to be tested individually.

This manner of testing is more dangerous, painful and time-consuming. One has to be very careful when testing small children. Some patients can go into anaphylactic shock due to the introduction of extremely allergic items into the body. The painful procedure can cause soreness for several days. The patient must wait for a few days or weeks between tests because only one set of allergens can be tested at a time. This method is not very effective in identifying allergies to foods unless you are extremely sensitive to them. Mild allergies are easily missed. Mild allergies can become severe with repeated and prolonged exposures to them over a period of time.

9. INTRADERMAL TEST

The intradermal test is considered to be more accurate for food allergies than a plain scratch test. The name comes from the fact that a small portion of the extract of the allergen is injected intradermally, between the superficial layers of skin. Many people who show no reaction to the dermal or scratch type of testing show positive results when the same allergens are applied intradermally. As in scratch tests, some patients can go into anaphylactic shock when extremely allergic items are injected into the body. The painful procedure can cause soreness for several days. The patient must wait a few days or weeks between tests, because only one set of allergens can be tested at a time.

10. RADIOALLERGOSORBANT TEST (RAST)

A sample of your blood is tested for antibodies. The radioallergosorbant test or RAST measures IgE antibodies in blood serum by radioimmunoassay and identifies specific allergens causing allergic reactions.

11. ELISA

Another blood serum test for allergies is called the "ELISA" (enzyme-linked immunosorbent assay) test. In this test, blood serum is tested for various immunoglobulin and their concentrations. Elisa can identify an antibody or antigen. The amount of antigen or antibody in the serum sample can be measured using this technique. This method is safe, sensitive, and simple to perform and provides reproducible results. For this test to show some positive results the patient must be exposed to particular foods within a certain amount of time. If the patient has never been exposed to certain foods, the test results may be unsatisfactory.

12. SUBLINGUAL TEST

Another prevalent allergy test, which is used by clinical ecologists and some nutritionists, is called a sublingual test. It involves the putting a tiny amount of allergen extract under the tongue. Then the response of the person is observed. If the test is positive, symptoms may appear very rapidly. The symptoms may include fast heart beats, increased breathing, dramatic mental and behavioral reactions in addition to physical reactions.

Applied kinesiologists and chiropractors use this same sublingual testing to test food allergens. A tiny amount of the food substance is placed under the tongue, and the patient is checked for weakness of predetermined strong muscle.

13. FOOD CHALLENGE

This is perhaps the oldest method for testing food allergies. The person is asked to abstain from eating the suspected allergic food for three to four days and then eating these to watch for symptoms. After the offending foods are identified, a diet is recommended by the allergist.

14. PULSE TESTING

Pulse testing is another simple way of determining food allergy. This test was developed by Arthur Coca M.D., in the 1950's. Research has shown that if you are allergic to something and you eat it, your pulse rate speeds up or slows down depending on the allergen's effect on sympathetic or parasympathetic nervous system. If it affects the sympathetic, pulse will speed up. If it affects parasympathetic, pulse will slow down.

Step 1: Establish your base line pulse by counting pedal pulse at the ankle or radial pulse at the wrist for a full minute.

Step 2: Put a small portion of the suspected allergen in a test tube and place it in the person's (child's) energy field (for example, place the test tube inside the socks, diaper, underpants, or under shirt, etc. for two minutes). Do not let the child eat the substance. The body contact with the substance will send the signal to the brain, which will send a signal through the sympathetic and parasympathetic nervous system to the rest of the body.

Step 3: Retake the pulse with the allergen still in the energy field. An increase in pulse rate of 10% or more or decreased of 10% is considered an allergic reaction. The greater the degree of allergy the greater the difference in the pulse rate.

This test is useful to test food allergies as well as environmental allergens such as fabrics, chemicals, insects, drugs, etc. Make sure the allergen is inside the test tube with a lid.

15. THE ELIMINATION DIET

The elimination diet, which was developed by Dr. Albert H. Rowe of Oakland, California, consists of a very limited diet that must be followed for a period long enough to determine whether or not any of the foods included in it are responsible for the allergic symptoms. If a fruit allergy is suspected, for example, all fruits are eliminated from the diet for a specific period, which may vary from a few days to several weeks, depending on the severity of the symptoms. For patients who have suffered allergic symptoms over a period of several years, it is sometimes necessary to abstain from the offending foods for several weeks before the symptoms subside. Therefore, the importance of adhering strictly to the diet during the diagnostic period is very important. When the patient has been free of symptoms for a specific period, other foods are added, one at a time, until a normal diet is attained. This may not be very convenient for young children.

16. ROTATION DIET

Another way to test for food allergy is through a "rotation diet," in which a different group of food is consumed every day for a week. In this method seven groups of food are consumed each week, with something different each day. The rotation starts again the following Monday. This way, reactions to any group can be traced and can be eliminated.

All of these diets work better for people who are less reactive. The inherent danger in any of these methods is clear: If you are highly allergic to a certain food you can become very sick if you eat that item during testing even if you have not touched it for years.

17. PEAK FLOW METER

A peak flow meter is a simple, portable, inexpensive device that measures the air flow. A peak flow meter can help you determine if your breathing function is normal or not and helps you monitor your asthma. With asthma, sometimes you may feel your breathing is fine, but when you measure it with a peak flow meter, your lung function is slightly decreased. This helps you to understand the pattern of your asthma and helps you manage better.

After taking a deep breath, you blow into the peek flow meter quickly and forcefully, and the resulting peak flow reading indicates how difficult it is to expell the air out of your lungs. A peak flow meter can be used to determine the following:

a. The severity of asthma;

b. Your response to treatment during an acute asthma episode;

c. The progress of treatment in chronic asthma cases;

d. The lung function on a daily basis without going through expensive testing procedures;

e. To detect the level of lung function when exposed to known allergens: you can write down peak flow meter readings before and after exposure to allergens such as foods, drinks, dust mites, irritants such as cigarette smoke, exercise or disturbing emotional events.

Asthma is usually worse at night, although some patients sleep through the night unaware of lower peak flow levels. During sleep, normally there is a decrease in the amount of oxygen in the blood and this drop in oxygen may happen more often and last longer in people with asthma. You do not have to wake up at night to use the meter; simply compare your morning reading with your reading the night before to determine the degree of night asthma. A decrease of 15% or greater from the previous night's measurement may indicate nocturnal asthma. Peak flow readings fall before the symptoms of asthma are otherwise noticed. The earlier a warning sign is detected, the sooner the problem can be addressed.

HOW TO USE A PEAK FLOW METER

There are several steps to properly using a peak flow meter. You should blow hard on the meter to get the best reading possible, and repeat this attempt three times. Record the best of three trials. All three measurements should be about the same to show that a good effort was made each time. This is especially important when parents are evaluating their child's asthma.

Follow these general steps when using a peak flow meter:

- Make sure the device reads zero or is at base level.
- Take the reading in standing position if possible.
- Place the meter in your mouth and close your lips around the mouthpiece.
- Take a full deep breath.
- Blow out as hard and as fast as possible (one to two seconds).
- Do not cough or let your tongue block the mouthpiece.
- Write down the value obtained.
- Repeat the process two additional times, and record the highest of the three numbers in your chart.

It is also helpful to record readings before and after using inhaled bronchodilator if you are using it. Write all the readings each morning and night. Graphs for plotting peak flow readings often come with the devices and can be photocopied for repeated use. Take it to your doctor on each visit. Your doctor can gain a great deal of information by reviewing these readings. This also will help you to gain a better understanding of your lung function.

Other Types of Allergy Testing

18. LIKE CURES LIKE

There are other allergy testing and treatments in practice. Homeopaths believe that if an allergen is introduced to the patient in minute concentrations at various times, the patient can build up enough antibodies toward that particular antigen. Eventually, the patient's violent reactions to that particular substance may reduce in intensity. In some cases, reactions may subside completely and the patient can use or consume the item without any adverse reaction.

All of the above methods work on a certain percentage of people. Everything may not work on everybody. One must find what test is best for one.

NAET Treatments During Pregnancy

I was treated with NAET during my first pregnancy, with amazing results. My chronic rhinitis of five years was resolved in four treatments. I decided to learn this technique to be able to provide myself, my family and my patients with a comprehensive treatment for allergies. Within a few days of NAET Basic Seminar I was able to treat myself for an acute shoulder pain and my son for a sudden cough, both resulted from eating allergic foods. NAET is a revolutionary means of evaluating and treating allergies painlessly, without risk. This is definitely going to be THE Medicine of the FUTURE!

NAET Sp: Gracie Lyons, M.D.

Phoenix, AZ

5

DIAGNOSIS OF ASTHMA

A detailed clinical history is the best diagnostic tool for any medical condition. It is extremely important for the patient, his/her parents or guardians to cooperate with the physician/NAET specialist in giving all possible information to the doctor in order to obtain the best results. It is my hope that this chapter will help bring about a clearer understanding between NAET specialists and their patients, because in order to obtain the most satisfactory results, both parties must work together as a team. Your NAET specialist's office may ask you to complete a relevant questionnaire during your first appointment. It is important to provide as accurate a history as possible.

STEPS TO DIAGNOSE ASTHMA

Steps to establish the diagnosis of asthma should consist of the following information about the patient.

1. General data sheet
2. Chief complaints
3. A detailed medical history

A detailed medical history should include the following information: presenting symptoms, pattern of symptoms, present medical history, frequency and severity of present symptoms (severity of the attacks, number of attacks by day, week, month, etc., number and frequency of hospitalizations, emergency room visits, response to medication, etc.), past medical history, personal health history, developmental history of the disease, prenatal history, growth and developmental history of the person, social history, behaviors, habits, occupation, hobbies, family history of asthma or allergies, precipitating or aggravating factors (effect of weather-change, exercise intolerance, change in living environment, job environment, etc.), short and long term goals expected from NAET treatments.

4. Has the patient been seen by pulmonologists prior to this visit, if so, give the name and address of the pulmonologist. Information also should be collected about current pharmacological therapies, medications, herbs, nutritional supplements, dietary history, other therapies received in the past or currently receiving, information on radiolological and other diagnostic evaluations. Previous medical records from other medical facilities should be requested with the patient's consent if that is necessary to evaluate the patient's present health condition.

5. Impact of asthma on patient and family, assessment of patient's and family's perception of disease, information about family support or other support while going through the treatment also should be gathered.

6. The knowledge of the patient and family and/or caretakers on how to manage the asthma, exacerbations, and complications also should be noted.

7. Informed consent must be signed by the patient or gurdian giving permission to the NAET specialist to provide the appropriate NAET treatment using his/her expertise to help with the presenting condition.

GENERAL DATA SHEET

Gathering the patient's medical and related personal data is essential to understand the patient's background. This data sheet should contain the following information: age, gender, marital status, job situation, work address, home address, telephone numbers, other identifying information, and a next of kin to contact in emergency.

Review of personal data will help the NAET specialist to understand the patient better: Is the patient a child/ under-age? A student? A mature adult? Employed or unemployed? Disabled due to illness? Capable of taking care of his/her needs, or dependent? Residential address, work address and job situation will help the NAET sp to understand the living and working environments.

CHIEF COMPLAINTS

Shortness of breath, the onset, intensity and duration.

If the patient is able, he/she is asked to describe the chief complaint in his/her own words. An asthma patient may present with the symptoms of shortness of breath, cough, wheezing, and mucus production in the throat. The intensity of the symptoms and duration of the present incident will be varied.

[The reason for such NAET symptom evaluation is as follows: The patient may have encountered a certain allergen that was capable of causing energy disturbances in the lung meridian, large intestine meridian, stomach meridian, spleen meridian, kidney meridian, urinary bladder meridian, liver meridian, gallbladder meridian and cental meridian, etc. (Read Chapter 7) giving rise to pathological symptoms evidenced by cough, wheezing, shortness of breath, and mucus production.]

PATTERN OF SYMPTOMS

The question should be asked about the pattern of frequency of occurrence of the attacks. Asthma may occur as seasonal or perennial, or both. The occurrence of asthmatic attacks will be episodic or continual, or both. The first onset of asthma also varies largely in different people from infancy to any age depending on many factors. Some people suffer from asthma only during the day and some may suffer only at night. Some people get asthma daily, some may get once a week and yet some may get only once a month or once a year. Some may get any time during the day and some get only at night or early morning and some are awakened in the middle of the night or early morning hours. We see all these variations.

[NAET evaluation: There are many reasons for these huge variations in different manifestations in different people. Often an asthmatic patient is sensitive to certain foods. If symptoms occur only on specific days of the week, they are probably due to something contacted or eaten on that particular day. Although foods may be a contributing factor, if the symptoms occur only at specific times of the year, the trouble most likely is due to something that is predominant around the patient at that time; for example: a particular grass pollen or flower pollen in the air may be the cause. Man has a natural tolerance for food that prevents the manifestation of asthma until one saturates the body with the particular allergic food or until the pollen sensitivity adds sufficient allergens to throw the body into an imbalance. The time of day when the attacks occur is also of importance in determining the cause of an asthmatic manifestation. If it always occurs before mealtime, low blood sugar may be a possible cause. If it occurs after meals, an allergy to something in the meal should be suspected. If it occurs regularly at bedtime, the toothbrush, toothpaste, mouth wash, makeup remover, night cream, night attire, etc., may be suspected. If it occurs regularly at night, it is quite likely that there is something in the bedroom that is aggravating the condition. It may be that the patient is sensitive to: feathers in the pillow, comforter, bed frame, mattress, wood cabinets, marble floors, carpets, side tables, end tables, bed sheets, pillows, pillow cases, detergents used in washing clothes, indoor plants, shrubs, trees, bed partner (an allergy to people), or grasses outside the patient's window.]

One of my patients suffered from severe asthmatic attacks at night as soon as he retired to bed. After spending a few minutes in bed, he regularly got up wheezing and spent the rest of the night sitting and wheezing without any sleep. He was found to be allergic to his wooden bed frame and expensive mattress that was made specifically to support his back.

The cause of disease can, at first, appear random. One young patient experienced regular attacks of rhinitis after he worked on his coloring books. The colors caused a severe allergic reaction. Another patient reacted similarly to the comic section of the newspaper.

A boy always developed a severe cough and later shortness of breath every day, halfway through sorting and wrapping up the local newspaper that he was assigned to distribute to his small community. He was found to be allergic to the newspaper ink and the paper itself.

A 30-year-old man suffered from asthmatic attacks every day at work and had to leave work early either to go to his doctor or home to rest. He worked in the financial deptartment. The cause was traced to his walnut desk at work where he spent every minute while working. He was advised to bring some woodshavings from the desk and we treated him with NAET. After he was treated for that particular desk, he no longer experienced the symptoms of asthma.

Another child had an allergic attack of sneezing, runny nose, mental irritability, and headaches on Saturdays. The cause was traced to an allergy to the shampoo her mother used to wash her hair on Friday afternoons.

No one has any explanation to why certain bodies react towards some things in certain way. An item may be absolutely harmless to one person and completely disastrous to the sensitive person.

PRESENT HISTORY

A careful medical history, and appropriate NTTs (Nambudripad's Testing Techniques include: Physical examination, pulmonary function tests, kinesiological tests and other relevant diagnostic studies) will provide the information needed to ensure a correct diagnosis of asthma. Some typical preliminary questions should include the following format of questioning.

When did your or your child's first symptom of asthma occur?

Did you notice your or your child's asthma as an infant or child, or during adolescence?

Did it occur after going through a certain procedure? For example, did it occur for the first time after a dental procedure, like applying braces or filling a cavity?

Did it happen after the first antibiotic treatment?

Did it happen after installing a water filter?

Did it happen after you started sleeping on a waterbed?

Did it happen after receiving a birthday present? A tricycle, a pearl necklace, a cotton summer dress? A hair dryer?

Did it occur after a booster dose of immunization?

Did it happen after putting in a lawn?

Did it happen after putting in a flower bed?

Did it happen after putting in a vegetable garden?

Did it happen after picking fruits from a tree?

Did it happen after working in the vegetable or fruit garden?

Did it happen after putting fertilizer on the plants?

Did it happen after spraying insecticides or pesticides to the plants in your garden?

Did it happen after spraying insecticides or pesticides to the plants in your neighborhood by the city?

Did it happen after eating vegetables and fruits from your garden?

Did it happen after you took a walk in the park?

Did your asthma begin after an insect bite?

Next, the doctor will want to know the circumstances surrounding and/or immediately preceding the first symptoms. Typical questions will include:

Did you change your or the child's diet or put him/her on a special diet?

Did you or he/she eat something that hadn't been eaten recently, perhaps for two or three months?

Did you eat or feed your child one type of food repeatedly, say, every day?

Did the asthmatic symptoms follow a childhood illness, (whooping cough, measles, chicken pox, diphtheria) or any immunization for such an illness?

Did your asthma follow some other illness such as influenza, pneumonia, a viral infection, bacterial infection, parasitic infestation, or a treatment program for any of these?

Did your asthma follow a major operation?

Did the asthma begin after your vacation to an island, to another country?

Did the asthma begin after camping in a cold, damp, camp ground? After an earthquake? After living through a tornado?

Did your asthma begin after wearing dry-cleaned clothes?

Did your asthma begin after walking in the rain?

Did your asthma begin after spraying pesticides in your neighborhood? Or walking in the park where the pesticide was sprayed earlier?

Did your asthma begin after eating a special food?

Did your asthma begin after using a special chemical to clean your carpet?

Did your asthma begin after getting a new car?

Did your asthma begin after bringing new furniture into the house?

Did your asthma begin after visiting a cigarette-smoke-filled casino?

Did your asthma begin after taking a course of antibiotics?

Did your asthma begin after starting a new vitamin supplement?

Did your asthma begin after going through a detoxification program?

Did your asthma begin after receiving other therapy, say for arthritis? Kidney dialysis? Blood transfusion? Dental work?

Did your asthma begin after an auto accident? Any other accident?

Did your asthma begin after receiving traumatic news?

Did your asthma begin after starting a new exercise program?

Did your asthma begin with any emotional trauma, like the house burning down during a wild fire, etc?

Did your asthma begin after the loss of a loved one?

Did your asthma begin after the loss of a pet?

Did your asthma begin after the loss of a toy?

Did your asthma begin with sadness?

Did your asthma begin with grief?

Did your asthma begin with guilt?

Did your asthma begin with frustration? Embarrassment? Shame?

Did your asthma begin with any stress, like loss of job, divorce, etc?

Any one of these factors can be responsible for triggering an asthma attack or precipitate the noticeable symptoms of an asthmatic condition. Therefore, it is very important for an NAET doctor to obtain full and accurate answers when taking the patient's medical history.

Present Symptoms

The NAET specialist will gather information about the frequency of asthma and the severity of the attacks in the patient's own words.

How often do you get asthma? ______________________

Daily (how many times?)______________________

Every other day_____________Once a week __________

Once a month ______________________

Once a year ______________________

After certain activities only ______________________

How long does an attack last? ______________________

Do you take any medication? Yes [ ] No [ ]

If you marked yes, please list your medications ______

____

Do you get relief after medication? Yes [ ] No [ ]

If so within how many minutes? ________________

Do you go to the emergency room to get relief? Yes [ ] No [ ]

How many times have you received emergency care for your asthma during this week? ______________________

Last month?______________________

Last 3 months? ______________________

Last 6 months? ______________________

Last 12 months______________________

The information should be obtained in the following areas:

Cough-productive: Yes [ ] No [ ]

Nonproductive: Yes [ ] No [ ]

Worse at night: Yes [ ] No [ ]

Worse during the day: Yes [ ] No [ ]

Recurrent wheezing, shortness of breath, chest tightness:

During the day: Yes [ ] No [ ]

During nights: Yes [ ] No [ ]

Before meals: Yes [ ] No [ ]

After meals: Yes [ ] No [ ]

After any activity: Yes [ ] No [ ]

If so, list the activity________________________________.

Other Factors Causing Asthmatic Symptoms

- Viral infection.
- Vocal cord dysfunction.
- Sinusitis, hay-fever, or rhinitis.
- Nasal polyp, gastroesophageal reflex disorders, or vocal cord anomaly.
- Enlarged glands, lymph nodes, growth, tumors and cancers.
- Cystic fibrosis, pulmonary embolism, and laryngeal dysfunction.
- Bronchopulmonary spasm, dysplacia, congestive cardiac failure.
- Cough due to other reasons: heart diseases, and chronic obstructive pulmonary diseases.

- Mechanical obstruction in the airways, aspiration of food or drinks, bronchospasm due to foreign body in the air way.
- Drug sensitivity and allergies.

PAST MEDICAL HISTORY

It is important to review the past medical history. History of development of asthma, previous treatments, age of first onset, frequency of occurrences, number of hospital admissions, emergency room visits, etc. should be obtained. History of any previous respiratory tract infections or diseases causing scars or fibrosis of the airways should be noted e.g. tuberculosis, bronchitis, pneumonia, abscess in the lung, bronchopulmonary dysplasia, exposure to secondary cigarette smoke from parents or caretakers, long term exposure to any other smoke, (breathing the smoke from the World Trade Center disaster, or the smoke from a wildfire in California), etc. should be noted.

If the patient has done any previous diagnosistic studies, or treatment at another facility, copies of the reports, treatment records, medication history, and progress reports from them should be requested. Also a record of any history of allergic symptoms in the patient should be made. The patient will be asked if he ever suffered from asthma, emphysema, rhinitis, sinusitis, frequent lung infections, or hay fever, ever suffered from hives, reacted to a serum injection (such as tetanus antitoxin, DPT), or experienced any skin trouble, whether the patient was unable to eat certain foods as a child or any time during his/her life, complained of repeated headaches, shortness of breath, dyspepsia, indigestion, joint pains, mood swings, bothered by weather changes, humidity, became restless or short of breath in the warm shower, got short of breath in high altitudes, bothered by extreme weathers like cold or heat, throat closing-like sensation caused by ice cream, frequent upper respiratory infections, or any other conditions where an allergy might have been a contributing factor for the asthma.

PERSONAL HEALTH HISTORY

Characteristics of home including age, location, cooling and heating system, wood burning stove, humidifier, carpeting over concrete, presence of molds, or mildew, characteristics of rooms where patient spends time: e.g., bedroom, and living room with attention to bedding, floor covering, stuffed furniture, picture frames, fireplace, indoor plants, animals, outdoor plants, any vines, trees, shrubs growing near the bedroom window, any unclean old spa or swimming pool near the bedroom, or any collection of junk outside the bedroom causing molds and mildew to grow. Also questions about any smell in or around the house should be asked. Smells from cooking, baking, coffee brewing, herbal concoctions, and other smells including perfume, aftershave lotion, shampoo, body lotion, smoking (patient and others in home or day care, workplace, and school surroundings) etc. which can trigger asthma in some people.

Other impeding factors such as peer pressure, fear from different sorts, substance abuse, gang involvements, cult involvements, etc. may trigger asthma in some people.

Questions also should be asked about the level of education completed, past or present employment (if employed, characteristics of work environment), family support, social support, or other support.

DEVELOPMENTAL HISTORY OF THE DISEASE

History of early life and developmental information through the years should be obtained if available. Many patients react violently to house dust, different types of furniture, polishes, house plants, tap water and purified water. Most of the city water suppliers change the water chemicals once or twice a year. People with chemical allergies may get asthma and other respiratory troubles if they inhale or ingest the same chemicals over and over for a period of time. Some patients who live near any chemical factories, factories that generate pesticides, insecticides, radioactive materials, living near electric circuits, environmental and chemical waste dumping areas, refuse dumps, cotton fields, gradually develop asthma over a period of time due to overexposure to the toxins and toxic wastes. If a person is allergic to radiation (computer, television, X-ray radiation, microwave radiation, etc.), eventually he/she can develop asthma. People living near a park (exposure to pesticides), working in a furniture factory (exposure to pesticides and heavy metals, PBDE - polybrominated diphenyl - a fire retardant chemical used in furniture making), working in a swimming pool supply, working with lead, silica, etc., working in pest control companies, working in fabric companies, people in sewing business are prone to get upper respiratory disorders and asthma. If the patient is a child, it is very important to get the complete prenatal history, growth and developnmental history.

PRENATAL HISTORY

Information on all these issues: socio-economic factors; exposures to substance abuse, heavy metal poisoning, coffee, alcohol, chemical toxins, carbon monoxide poisoning, bacterial toxins; emotional traumas during fetal development or later years; birth records including birth weight and APGAR scores.

Growth and Developmental History

ILLNESSES DURING EARLY INFANCY

Presence of any of these symptoms in infancy or childhood will confirm the inherted allergic tendency even though it was not manifested as asthma at that time. Mark it with a check in the appropriate column.

[ ] Colic

[ ] Constipation

[ ] Diarrhea

[ ] Feeding problem

[ ] Excessive vomiting

[ ] Excessive white coating on the tongue

[ ] Excessive crying

[ ] Poor sleep

[ ] Disturbed sleep

[ ] Frequent ear infection

[ ] Frequent fever

[ ] Immunizations

[ ] Response to the immunizations

[ ] Common childhood diseases like measles, chickenpox, mumps, strep-throat, etc.

[ ] Any other unusual events (fire in the house, accidents, earthquakes, smoke inhalation, carbon monoxide poison ing, death in the family, a new pet, etc).

DEVELOPMENTAL MILESTONES

Mark with a check in the appropriate column. Write the age, year, frequency, or number of times, if applicable.

⇒ AGE OF THE CHILD

[ ] Walked alone________________

[ ] Talked ________________

[ ] Toilet trained for bladder and bowel ________________

[ ] Enrolled in school ________________

⇒ MEDICAL HISTORY OF EARLY LIFE

[ ] Surgeries________________

[ ] Hospitalizations ________________

[ ] Diseases ________________

[ ] Allergies ________________

[ ] Frequent colds ________________

[ ] Fever ________________

[ ] Ear infections ________________

[ ] Asthma ________________

[ ] Hives ________________

[ ] Bronchitis ________________

[ ] Pneumonia ________________

[ ] Seizures ________________

[ ] Sinusitis ________________

[ ] Headaches ________________

[ ] Vomiting ________________________

[ ] Diarrhea ________________________

[ ] Current medication ________________

[ ] Any reaction to medication __________

[ ] Antibiotics and drugs taken __________

[ ] Parasitic infestation ________________

[ ] Visited other countries ______________

SOCIAL HISTORY

Learning: Grades at school, interaction between friends and teachers, interaction between family members, activities at school, phobias, and problems with discipline. (A child may not yet to manifest with obvious asthma symptoms, but allergies to things in his/her environment can cause the child have problems in any of these areas. Eventually such allergies can manifest in asthma).

Behaviors: Cooperative, uncooperative, disruptive and/or aggressive behaviors; overactive, restless, inattentive, day dreams; uncooperative with his/her peers and adults; incomplete or sloppy work (These also could be due to allergies to food additives and other chemicals).

Habits: Obsession, compulsion, frequent clearing of the throat, itching and picking nose, vomiting after meals, temper tantrums, depression, quietness, remain isolated and not playing with others, clinging to mother all the time (feelings of insecurity), restless leg syndrome (an allergy to food or something in the bed), unusual fears and fatigue.

Hobbies: Reading, golfing, tennis, walking in the park, horse-back riding, painting, etc.

Occupation: Students, writers, lawyers, doctors, bakers, cooks, managers in different areas, store keepers, beauticians, cleaners, gardeners, teachers, painters, road workers, field workers, factory workers, engineers, drivers, entertainers, etc.

No job is exempted from getting exposed to dangerous allergens. Potential allergens are hiding in unexpected places and any one of them can trigger an asthmatic attack in a sensitive person. Avoiding the allergen is not a permanent solution. Running away from a problem will not help us to solve the problem. One needs to face the problem and eliminate it. NAET treatments can eliminate the problems permanently.

FAMILY HISTORY

The medical history of the immediate relatives, mother, father, and siblings should be noted. The questions should be asked about history of asthma, emphysema, allergy, sinusitis, rhinitis, sinus surgeries, or nasal polyps in patient's immediate relatives. The same questions are asked about the patient's nonimmediate relatives: grandparents, aunts, uncles, brothers, sisters, cousins. A tendency to get sick or have allergies or asthma is not always inherited directly from the parents. It may skip generations or manifest in nieces or nephews rather than in direct descendants.

The inquiry should include not only about asthma and respiratory illnesses, but other allergy-related health disorders like alcoholism, autoimmune disorders, drug abuse, smoking, eating disorders, addictive behaviors, mental disorders, other health disorders. The careful NAET specialist will also determine whether or not diseases such as tuberculosis, cancer, heart disease, diabetes, rheumatic or glandular disorders exist, or have ever occurred in the patient's family history.

All of these facts help give the NAET specialist a complete picture of the hereditary characteristics of the patient. An allergy may be manifested differently in different people, even if it is familial. As example, parents may have had cancer or rheumatism, but the child can manifest that inheritance as asthma.

Complicating Factors

A single allergen, or a group of allergens, or an incident may have triggered the asthma in a patient. But it usually does not end there. More allergens from the environment will begin to affect the weakened immune system of the victim. He/she may have been allergic to a large group of substances in the surroundings but until an allergen triggered a major reaction, others were kept under control by the body's natural defense. When the first major allergen sets forth the initiative, a chain reaction will begin with all other allergens causing cascades of reactions creating more complication for the sufferer. Such people can suffer from asthma many times a day in varying degrees and intensities, taking a long time to respond to any medication or therapy. Aggravating factors should be avoided or the reaction between the body and the allergens should be eliminated (via NAET treatments) before they can show any response to the medication or therapy. Some of the commonly seen allergens which can act like triggers can be seen in the following lists.

SYMPTOMS OCCUR OR WORSEN:

After Inhaling Substances

Inhaling pollens while walking in the park when the pollen count is high; inhaling after-shave lotions, airborne chemicals, benzene, body lotions, body soap, chemical smells from city water, cigarette smoke, cleansing agents, colognes, cooking smells, cosmetic products, cut grass smell, dental materials, detergents, diesel, dust, exhausts, fabric softeners, fertilizers, fireplace smoke, flowers, food seasoning smell, formaldehyde, frying food smell, fungicides, gasoline, hair products, hair sprays, herbal supplements, herbicides, hospital supplies (smell from oxygen tubes, rubber or plastic catheters, surgical instruments, surgical sutures, hospital cleaning agents, disinfectants, anesthetics, drugs), house cleaning chemicals, house dust, and dust mites, hydrocarbons, insects (cockroach, bee, fly, flea, ants, etc.), insecticide sprays, laboratory chemicals, leather smell, massage oils, molds and mildews, fungus, new car smell, newspaper ink, newspaper, paper products, outdoor allergens (tree pollens, trees, shrubs, weeds, flowers, grass, fibers floating in the air from cotton pods when they mature before picking them from the trees, lint wastage from cotton mills and other fabric mills, fumes from chemical factories, silica dust from silica factory, radioactive waste or fallout from the storage or factory, paint fumes, etc.), perfumes, personal protective equipment (latex gloves, masks), pesticides, plastic products, polishes, prescription drugs, shampoo, smell from animals and animal products, smell from cat litter, smell from coffee brewing, smell from candle burning, smell from food, smell from popcorn, smell from paint fumes, smell from soiled baby-diaper, smell of body secretions (saliva, semen, vaginal discharge, sputum, sweat, bad breath, menstrual blood, stool, urine, body odor), smell from room fresheners, soap, sugar cane burning smoke, wild fire burning smoke, synthetic fabrics, tobacco smoke, varnishes, vitamins, wood burning smoke, wood furniture, wood polish.

After Ingesting any Meal

Alcoholic drinks, antibiotics (in meat, milk, other products), artificial food coloring, beans, bell pepper, beverages, cactus, carob, chewing gums, chicken, chocolate, cinnamon, condiments, cooked food, cooking sprays, corn, dried fruits, drinking water, drinks, drugs (aspirin, beta-blockers, nonsteroidal anti-inflammatory drugs, cardiac, analgesics, topicals, and others), egg plant, eggs, fish, food additives, food preservatives, fruits, garlic, grains, grapes, hormone supplements, meat, medication, melons, mushroom, nutmeg, nuts, onion, pain relieving medication, pineapple, potato, prenatal vitamins, prepackaged food, protein drinks, rain water, raisins, salt, sea salt, sea water, soy products, special diets, spices, sugar, sulfites, thyroid medication, tomato, uncooked food, vegetables, vitamins, weight loss diets, water chemicals, water filter salts, wheat, and yeast.

When Contacted Certain Substances

Acetate, acrylic, animal dander, animal epithelial, bathroom slippers, bed linen, animals and animals with fur or feathers, bed room furniture, books, carpets, ceramic cups, ceramic tiles, chair, cleaning chemicals, cockroach, coloring books, coloring equipments, cooking pans, cotton fabrics, crayons, crib toys, curtains, dental equipment, dental filling materials, dentures, dining table, dishwashing soap, down comforter, drapes, elastics, electronic toys, exercising equipments, feather pillows, hair brush, hair dryer, heavy metals, highlighters, house plants in the bed room, house-dust mites, interior decorating materials, jewelry, kitchen cleaning materials like scrubbers, latex products, liquid paper, mattress, mercury, mouth wash, night blooming plants if the window is left open, night wear clothes, office products, other fabrics, paintings, pencils, pens, personal hygiene products, pillows, plastic sheets, plastic toys, prosthesis, pajama, reading books, remote control for the TV, rubber, sanitary napkins, school bag, school desk, school work material, shoe, silverware, socks, stuffed toys, table cloth, table mat, tampons, tap water, teflon coating on the pans, tennis ball, tennis racket, the night air, toothbrush, toothpaste, underwear, upholstered furniture, wall paint, wall picture, wall poster, water bed, work material, and wristwatch.

After Injecting Anything into the Body

Allergy shots, insulin shots, vitamin shots, hormone shots, vaccinations, immunizations, insect bites, mosquito bites, bee stings, stung by corals, shellfish, sea urchins, dog bites, cat scratches, animal bites of other sources, bitten by ticks, fleas, flies, ants, etc.

After Contacting Infectious Agents

After exposure to virus, bacteria, parasite, either exposed through eating uncooked or spoiled foods or lived in closed contact with people with viral, bacterial infections, parasitical infestation, molds, mildews, fungi, decayed materials, or suffering from other contagious diseases. Sometimes infections can spread by contacting the materials handled by the suffering person: utensils, silverware, body secretions, sharing the same toilet, bath towels, etc.

After Exposing to Extreme Weather Conditions

Heat, cold, playing in the snow, dryness, dampness, humid conditions, fog, wind, damp-heat, damp-cold, draughts, cold air from air conditioner, etc.

After Exposure to Occupational Hazards

Tobacco smoke, strong odors, air pollutants, occupational chemicals, dusts particles, cleaning chemicals, noises, airplane fuel or exhaust, airplane noises, vapors and gases.

After Experiencing Emotional Traumas

After facing events leading to excessive laughing, excessive crying, sadness, grief, frustration, betrayal, depression, aggression, fear, anger, diagnosed with an unexpected new disease such as cancer, diagnostic testing procedures, surgery, changing homes, places, moving to another country, new friends, new life experiences, new additions to the family by birth or marriage, financial loss, human loss, material loss, post traumatic stress disorders, etc.

Sudden Change in Living Environments

Molds, mildews, fungi, decayed materials in the new environments, moving home, buying new home, renovation or construction of the home, vacation, changing jobs, changing states, country, new life-style, changing schools, starting a new school, starting a new career, starting a new life, etc.

When Going Through Hormonal Changes or Disturbances

Changes in the status of menses, pregnancy, delivery, thyroid imbalances, pituitary imbalances, people who suffer from gastroesophageal reflex disorders, congestive heart failure, heart diseases, kidney disorders, people on dialysis, etc.

During or After Exercise

During exercise, production of endorphins, enkaphalins, neurotransmitters, and certain hormones like pheromones, etc., are stimulated. If the patient is allergic to these secretions they can trigger asthma in sensitive people. Some people get sinus congestion, and shortness of breath or even asthma during sexual intimacy. That is because the patient may be allergic to pheromones produced by the body during sexual intimacy.

Role of NAET Specialist

1. Short Term Goal of NAET in Asthmatics

II. Long Term Goals of NAET in Asthmatics

I. Short Term Goal of NAET in Asthmatics

1. Prevent Symptoms of Asthma

Prevent symptoms of asthma during the day and night (e.g.cough, shortness of breath, wheezing, post nasal drip, mucus in the throat, etc.) by treating the patient for NAET basic allergens. Two or three times a week treatment is advised initially in order to complete the treatment on the first 20 NAET basic allergens in order to provide the patient some early relief of asthma symptoms. Eighty percent of the asthma cases diminish their symptoms and reduce the need for asthma medications by the time they successfully complete treatments for 20 NAET basic allergens.

2. Improve Quality of Life

1. Avoid all known allergens until treated.
2. Continue all asthma medications and therapies as prescribed.
3. Increase the activity as tolerated.

II. Long Term Goals of NAET in Asthmatics

1 Maintain normal pulmonary function.

2 Maintain normal activity levels.

3 Prevent recurrent attacks of asthma.

4 Prevent exacerbations of asthma.

5 Minimize emergency room visits and hospitalizations.

6 Improve the quality of life.

7 Educate the patient, family or caretakers/assistants in asthma care.

1. Maintain Normal Pulmonary Function

Patient should be referred to a qualified pulmonologist for consultation if the patient is not seeing one already and co-management with pharmacotherapy in the initial stages of asthma care and to maintain pulmonary function record. It is very important to keep the asthma under control while going through NAET treatment. If the symptoms are kept under control, NAET works better. In milder cases, herbs and nutritional supplements might help control the asthma while going through NAET treatments.

Severe cases must seek appropriate pharmacotherapy to keep the symptoms under control until the allergens are treated and eliminated from your life.

2. Maintaining Normal Activity Levels

1. Encourage the patient to use a peak flow meter and monitor the asthma occurrences and intensities after any physical activities and adjust the activities accordingly.
2. Treat all known allergens through NAET.
3. Maintain a daily treatment log or journal.

3. Prevent Recurrent Asthmatic Attacks

1. The patient should be taught NAET self-testing.
2. The patient should be taught NAET asthma reducing points and teach them to use at the first sign of asthma symptoms.

4. Prevent Exacerbations of Asthma

The patient should be taught NAET self-balancing, and adivise them to do them daily, twice a day, until they are free of asthma.

5. Minimize E.R.visits or Hospitalizations

1. The patient should learn the acupressure emergency help points.

2. The patient should carry epi-pen and antihistamines all the time and never hesitate to use them when they are needed.

7. The patient should call 911 or seek emergency help immediately when needed in any acute situation.

6. Improve the Long-term Quality of Life

1. The patient should avoid all known allergens until treated with NAET.

2. Nutritional evaluation and supplementation to maintain adequate nutrition.

3. Follow-up with the NAET specialist regularly for the treat ments until the known allergens are treated.

4. After treating for all known allergens, continue follow-up visits with the NAET specialist in the following schedule:

a. Once a month for three months, once in three months for the first year, once in six months for the second year, and then once a year.

b. Follow-up with the pulmonologist: Once in six months for five years for complete evaluation of the pulmonary function. Then yearly check up should be enough provided you do not get any more asthma episodes.

7. Educate the patient and family

1. The family and caretakers should help the patient avoid the item from the patient's list of detected allergens until the patient is treated for them.

1. The family should be taught NAET self-testing.

2. The family should be taught NAET asthma reducing points and teach them to use at the first sign of asthma symptoms.

3. The family should be taught how to use epi-pen and antihistamines and help the patient to use if needed.

4. The family should call 911 or seek emergency help when needed in any acute situation.

Self-testing

The NAET sp should teach the patient self-testing using "O" Ring test, Finger-on-finger test, and Dynamometer testing. Family or the helper should also learn how to test for allergies using Neuro Muscular Sensitivity Testing.

Self-balancing

Acupressure self-balancing techniques are given with illustration in Chapter 9 for asthma. More acupressure therapeutic points for various disorders can be learnt from my book, "Living Pain Free" and can be purchased from www.amazon.com or from NAET website. The patient can easily learn to balance his/her body using these pressure points. According to Oriental medical theory, when the body is maintained at perfect balance, diseases or allergic reactions do not happen. The patient is encouraged to self-balance twice a day, upon awakening and before going to bed. The family or helper can also be taught to balance the patient using these asthma reducing acuhelp points.

Acupressure Emergency Help Points

Acupressure emergency help points are given with illustration in Chapter 9. Knowing how to use these Oriental medicine Cardio Pulmonary Resuscitation (CPR) points can help you overcome immediate emergencies and help you stay awake and alive until help arrives or until you are able to call for help or reach the nearest emergency room. The family or helper could also learn how to use these acupressure emergency resuscitation points.

Carry Epi-pen and Antihistamines

When one has a history of asthma, one does not know when one will react to some unsuspected allergen and get a severe reaction. To avoid any unexpected surprises, the patient should get a prescription from the pulmonologist for epi-pen and/or antihistamine and carry them at all the times and never hesitate to use them when they are needed. Patient should check the expiry date on the medication regularly and get a new prescription when the current ones are expired. The family should learn the proper administration of these drugs and use the epi-pen or the antihistamine appropriately on the patient if and when the need arises.

Advice to the family

NAET specialist should meet with the patient's family and caretakers or assistants in his/her care and educate them about the importance of understanding the signs, and symptoms of asthma and the possibility of sudden exacerbations if the patient comes in contact with any allergen. Family and caretakers should be taught to avoid the allergens from the patient's list of detected allergens until the patient is treated for them when the patient is nearby. If someone eats the allergen around the patient, he/she can react to it and trigger an asthmatic attack. So other family members should avoid the patient's allergens from being eaten or used when the patient is nearby. Family members need to be aware of the impact of the patient's sickness on the family, if he gets a sudden severe asthma and if he needs to go to the emergency room or hospital. If they learn to test and not to expose the patient to known allergens, they can avoid unwanted emergencies.

NUTRITIONAL EVALUATION

When someone has allergies to basic everyday foods, he/ she may not be absorbing the essential nutritients from the daily food. This malabsorption creates a huge nutritional deficiency in the patient. The NAET Basic treatments are made up of essential nutritients from one's daily diet. More detailed explanation about NAET Basic treatments is given in Chapter 8. After eliminating the allergy, the essential nutritients should be supplemented for faster recovery.

Evaluation of Activity

Importance of moderate amount of exercise cannot be stressed enough. Exercise is necessary to help improve the circulation in order to distribute the nutrients to different parts of the body. Improved circulation will also help eliminate the toxins from the body. Encourage the patient to add some mild exercise plan into the daily agenda. More on exercise is given in Chapter 10.

Follow-up with NAET

Follow-up with your NAET specialist regularly for treatments until the known allergens are treated and desensitized. The NAET Guidebook (available at www.amazon.com) is a very important and useful handbook to help you successfully complete the NAET treatments. After treating for all known allergens, continue follow-up visits with your NAET specialist in the following schedule: Once a month for three months, once in three months for the first year, once in six months for the second year, and then onwards once a year or as and when the need arises.

Patient should continue to maintain the daily log of foods eaten, foods not eaten but prepared by the patient, and any problems encountered while cooking or eating. Any unusual events happened to physical health or emotional health, any trips made to other cities, had to live through any disasters like earthquakes, tornado, flood, fire disaster, smoke inhalation, etc. should be recorded in the log and brought to the NAET doctor at each visit. The NAET sp will evaluate your physical and emotional responses to the events and if needed he/she will provide NAET to eliminate the effects of the trauma(s).

Follow-up with the pulmonologist

Patient should be seen by a pulmonologist for regular evaluaton as often as needed during the treatment phase. After completing the NAET program, patient should visit a pulmonologist one in six months for five years for complete evaluation of the pulmonary function. Patient should have a complete examination of all systems including respiratory system with a pulmonologist every six months to ensure the safety of the patient's health. Patient should refill the prescription for epi-pen and carry with them always at least for five years after completing NAET program. If the patient never had another asthma episode in five years following the completion of NAET treatment program, then the patient can discuss with his/her pulmonologist regarding the need for further carrying the epi-pen with him all the time. NAET specialist will not help you make that decision.

A SELF-EVALUATION FOR ASTHMA

Name____
Age_____________________________ Sex ____________________

Do you suffer from asthma? Any allergy? Or Allergy-related disorder? Below is an allergy-check list to help you evaluate yourself to see if you have any active or hidden allergies that might be causing your asthma. Please mark with a check where appropriate.

A sensible solution can be found if you can identify the source of your problem.

1. Please describe your chief problem in one sentence.

____

Please rate your symptoms on a scale of 0- 4: (0= no symptoms; 1= mild symptoms; 2= moderate symptoms; 3= severe symptoms; 4= extremely-severe)

II. Present History

1. How is your energy generally at these following hours?
6 am [ ], 8 am [ ], 10 am [ ], 12 noon [ ], 2 pm [ ], 4 pm [ ],
6 pm [ ], 8 pm [ ], 10 pm [ ], 12 am [ ], 2 am [ ], 4 am [ ]

2. How is your appetite? ______________[ ]
3. How is your digestion? ______________[ ]
4. How is your elimination? ____________[ ]
5. How is your sleep? _________________ [ ]
6. How is your mental clarity? __________[ ]
7. How is your general well-being? ____ [ ]
8. Have you seen another medical professional for your present complaints? Yes [ ] No [ ]

9. Have you been previously diagnosed with Asthma by another doctor? Yes [ ] No [ ]
10. Are you taking any medications now? Yes [ ] No [ ]

If you are taking any medication, please list them, the dosage and frequency ______________________________

MEDICAL DATA EVALUATION FORM

Name______________________________________
Age____________ Sex __________________________

1. Do you suffer from any of the following Symptoms?
   [ ]Cough
   [ ]Wheezing
   [ ]Shortness of breath
   [ ]Chest tightness
   [ ]Mucus production

2. List the characteristics of your asthma
   [ ]Perennial, [ ] seasonal, [ ] both
   [ ] Continual, [ ] episodic, [ ] both

3. Onset______________________________________

4. Duration/frequency ____________________________
   (number of days or nights, per week or month)
   [ ] Waking up night. If so, the approximate time————
   [ ] Waking up in the early morning hours ————

5. Viral respiratory infections

Yes [ ] No [ ]

6. Environmental allergens, indoor (e.g. mold, house-dust, dust-mite, cockroach, animal dander, or secretory products), and outdoor (e.g. pollen) ________________________________

7. Exercise-induced Yes [ ] No [ ]

8. Exercise-aggravated Yes [ ] No [ ]

9. Exposure to occupational /chemical allergens Yes [ ] No [ ]

10. Environmental changes (e.g. moving to new home; going on vacation; and/or alteration in workplace, work processes, or materials used). Explain ______________________________

____

11. Irritants (e.g., tobacco smoke, strong odors, air pollutants, occupational chemicals, dusts and particulates, vapors and gases). Explain__________________________________

12. Emotional factors (e.g., fear, anger, frustration, crying or laughing) ____

13. Drugs (e.g., Aspirin, beta-blockers, including eye drops non-steroidal anti-inflammatory drugs, and others)______________

14. Food, food additives, and preservatives (e.g., sulfites)

15. Changes in weather, exposure to cold air.

16. Endocrine factors (e.g., menses, pregnancy, thyroid disease)

17. Age of onset and diagnosis

18. History of previous respiratory illnesses (e.g., pneumonia, bronchitis, lung abscess, injury from smoking, secondary smoke)

Progress of disease [ ] better [ ] worse

19. Present treatment plan: describe: ___________________

____

20. Response _____________________________________

21. Patient/family education________________________
22. Advice given to handle emergencies __________________
____
____

23. In the past 12 months:

Have you had a sudden severe episode or recurrent episodes of coughing, wheezing (high-pitched whistling sounds when breathing out), or shortness of breath? [ ] Yes [ ] No

Have you had colds that "go to the chest" or take more than 10 days to get over? [ ] Yes [ ] No

[Have you had coughing, wheezing, or shortness of breath in certain places or when exposed to certain things)e.g., animals, tobacco, smoke, perfume)? [ ] Yes [ ] No

Have you used any medications/herbs that help you breathe better? If so how often? ________________________

Do you get relief from symptoms after medication? If so,

[ ] Partially [ ] Fully [ ] No relief

24. In the past four weeks, have you had coughing, wheezing, or shortness of breath? [ ] Yes [ ]No

If so, number of times __________________________

25. Have you experienced asthma symptoms at night?
[ ] Yes [ ] No

In the early morning? [ ] Yes [ ] No

After running [ ] Yes [ ] No

After moderate exercise [ ] Yes [ ] No

After other physical activity? [ ] Yes [ ] No

26. History of asthma, allergy, sinusitis, rhinitis, or nasal polyps in close relatives ________________________________

27. List of all known allergens________________________

____

28. Smoking - Patient and others in home or work or day care

____

29. Support from family or friends ___________________
30. Level of education completed ____________________
31. Employment (if employed, characteristics of work environment)____

32. How does this disease affect the family?_____________
33. Unexpected emergencies (E.R department, urgent care, hospitalization) __________________________________
34. Life-threatening exacerbations (e.g., intubation, intensive care unit admission) ______________________________
35. Number of days missed from school/work ____________
46. Limitation of activity, for school or work _____________
37. Nocturnal episodes needing attention from the family _____
38. Impact on family routines, and activities ______________
39. Economic impact ____________________________

PERCEPTION AND BELIEFS

1. Patient, parental, and spouse's or partner's knowl edge of asthma and belief in the chronicity of asthma and in the efficacy of treatment

2. Patient perception and beliefs regarding belief in the chronicity of asthma and in the efficacy of treatment

3. Ability of the patient and/or family in following instruct ions

4. Ability of patient and parents, spouse, or partner to cope with disease

5. Level of family support and patient's and parents', spouse's, or partner's capacity to recognize severity of an exacerbation

6. Economic resources

Environmental Allergies

At a time when food sensitivities, asthma, and environmental allergies in children are increasing at an alarming rate, NAET offers a safe, effective alternative to drug treatment that yields exceptional and lasting results.

Robert Sampson, M.D., FAACAP

Andover, MA (978) 474-9009

Shellfish Allergy

One young man had been afflicted with severe asthma every time he ate sea food. Because of his reactions to shellfish and crab meat, he had to eat non-seafood items when his family went to a traditional all-you-can-eat crab broil around Thanksgiving each year. After he received NAET clearing for seafood, I saw him at a family gathering about a month later and asked how his NAET treatment was holding up. He said, "I've been making up for ten years of lost time." I like to think of NAET as the ultimate technique for dealing with food allergies.

NAET Sp: Iris Prince, R.N.

Charlotte, North Carolina

6

Neuro Muscular Sensitivity Testing (NMST)

Neuro Muscular Sensitivity Testing (NMST) is one of the tools used by NAET specialists to detect imbalances in the body along with NTT. NTT will be described in detail in the following pages.

Neuromuscular sensitivity testing is slightly different from standard muscle response testing practiced by AK practitioners and various other practitioners of applied kinesiology. Whoever has studied NAET muscle response testing knows that this technique is different from all other existing muscle testing.

When the allergen's incompatible electromagnetic energy comes close to a person's energy field, repulsion takes place. Without recognizing this repulsive action, we frequently go near allergens (whether they are foods, drinks, chemicals, environmental substances, animals or humans) and interact with their energies. This energy disturbance produces energy blockages in the energy meridians creating disorganization in body functioning giving rise to various types of allergic reactions and diseases.

To prevent the allergen from causing further disarray, the brain sends messages to every cell in the body to reject it. The person will then experience some sort of physical, physiological, and/or psychological responses. This might include weak limbs, tiredness, aches, pains, insomnia, constipation, anger, depression, or other such unpleasant symptoms. The particular allergen, say, strawberry, might not be harmful to someone else but this person's brain perceives it as harmful and tries to remove it from its electromagnetic field.

Further changes can be noted in the person's neuromuscular sensitivity. When tested with an NMST procedure, this neuromuscular hyper or hypo sensitivity will show up as weakness in a previously tested strong muscle. When detecting such weakness, the NAET practitioner will have discovered the person's allergy to strawberry.

Allergy to Wool and Cigarette Smoke

I have had a lifetime of allergies, including asthma, hay fever, sinus problems and eczema. Two of my worst allergies were to wool and cigarette smoke. I had become so allergic to wool that I could not wear it or be around anyone who wore it without choking up, developing a headache, raspy throat, and often an asthmatic attack. Since Dr. Devi's treatment for wool, I am able to wear wool for the first time in many years without producing any unpleasant symptoms. Allergy to ciga-

rette smoke was crippling me socially. The treatment for cigarette smoke has given me more comfort socially since I don't have to isolate myself from friends. I don't know how to express my gratitude to Dr. Devi for discovering this new treatment method to eliminate allergies permanently.

Gene Fowler
Fullerton, CA

Tina, a nine-year-old girl, was undergoing treatment for asthma by NAET. She was treated for various foods and she was able to eat all of them without provoking an asthmatic attack. One day, her parents took her to a Chinese restaurant. When the food was brought to the table, she immediately whispered to her mother that she thought she was allergic to some of the food items on the plate and that she might become ill if she ate the food. The girl's mother ignored her and forced her to eat the food, saying that she had been treated for all of them. Before she finished eating, she had an asthmatic attack. The confused mother brought a sample of everything the child ate to the office next day. She was found to be allergic to the mixed vegetables that contained a great deal of cornstarch. She had not yet been treated for the corn. The nine-year-old was able to recognize the allergen before she ate it. She said her throat started itching as soon as the food was placed in front of her, giving her a clue that she might be allergic to something on the plate.

Your body has a way of telling you when you are in trouble. When you go near allergens, your brain will begin to produce various symptoms in your body in varying degrees, such as: an itchy throat, watery eyes, sneezing attacks, coughing spells, unexplained pain anywhere in the body, yawning, sudden tiredness, etc. If you learn to understand your brain and its clues closely you may be able to avoid many unpleasant events in your life including many serious health disorders. NMST is a good tool that can be used successfully to identify the same allergens. In this procedure, you will compare the strength of a strong muscle in your body (muscle from arm, leg, finger, neck, etc.) in the presence and absence of a suspected allergen. If a previously strong muscle tests weak in the presence of a substance, the substance is an allergen. If the substance was not able to elicit a weakness in the previously strong muscle, then the substance is not an allergen. NAET specialists use NMST to identify the presence of allergens around you.

NMST

(See illustrations of NMST on the following pages.)

NMST can be performed in the following ways:

1. Standard NMST can be done in standing, sitting or lying positions. You need two people to do this test: the person who is testing, the "tester," and the person being tested, the "subject."
2. The oval ring test can be used in testing yourself. This can also be used in testing a physically strong person. This requires two persons, as in standard NMST.
3. Surrogate testing can be used in testing an infant, an invalid person, a very strong or a very weak person, an animal, a plant or a tree. In this case, the surrogate's muscle is tested by the tester, and the subject maintains skin-to-skin contact with the surrogate while being tested and/or treated. The surrogate is not affected by the testing.

STANDARD NMST

Two people are required to perform standard NMST. The subject can be tested lying down, standing or sitting. The lying-down position is the most convenient for both the tester and the subject. It also achieves more accurate results.

Step 1: The subject lies on a firm surface with one arm raised (left arm in the picture below) 45-90 degrees to the body with the palm facing outward and the thumb facing toward the big toe.

Step 2: The tester stands at the subject's (right) side. The subject's right arm is kept to his/her side with the palm either kept open to the air, or in a loose fist. The fingers should not touch any material, fabric or any part of the table the arm is resting on. This can give wrong test results. The left arm of the subject is raised 45-90 degrees to the body. The tester's left palm is contacting the subject's left wrist (Figure 6-1).

Step 3: The tester, using the left arm, tries to push down on the subject's raised left arm toward the subject's left big toe. The subject resists the push with the arm muscle. The test muscle is called an "indicator muscle or predetermined muscle" or PDM for short. The PDM remains strong if the subject is well balanced at the time of testing. It is essential to test a strong PDM to get accurate results. Either the subject is not balanced, or the tester is performing the test improperly if the muscle or raised arm is weak and gives away under pressure without the presence of an allergen. For example, the tester might be trying to overpower the subject. The subject does not need to gather up strength from other muscles in the body to resist the tester. Only five to ten pounds of pressure needs to be applied on the

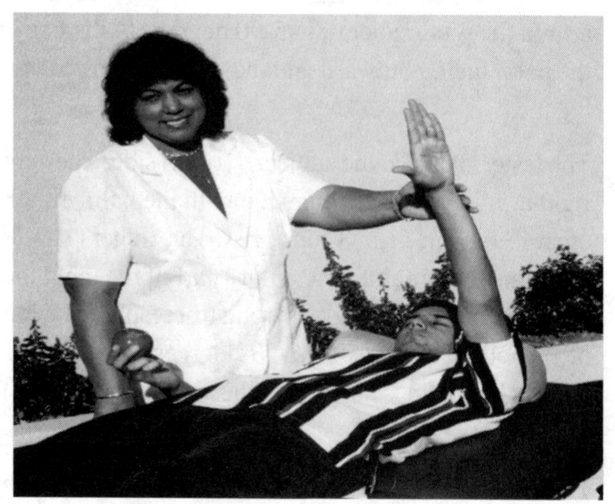

STANDARD NMST
FIGURE 6-1

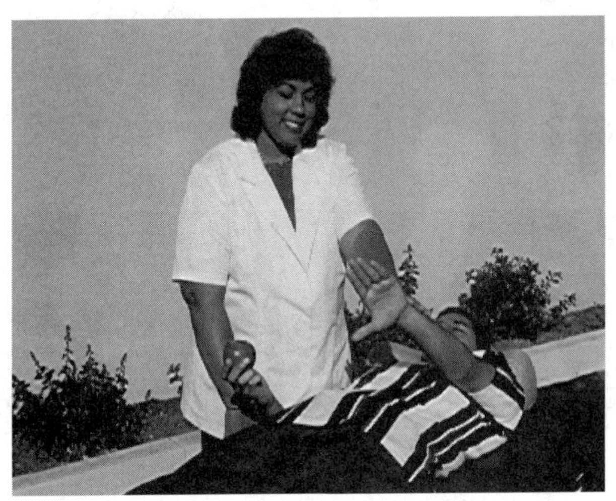

NMST WITH ALLERGEN
FIGURE 6-2

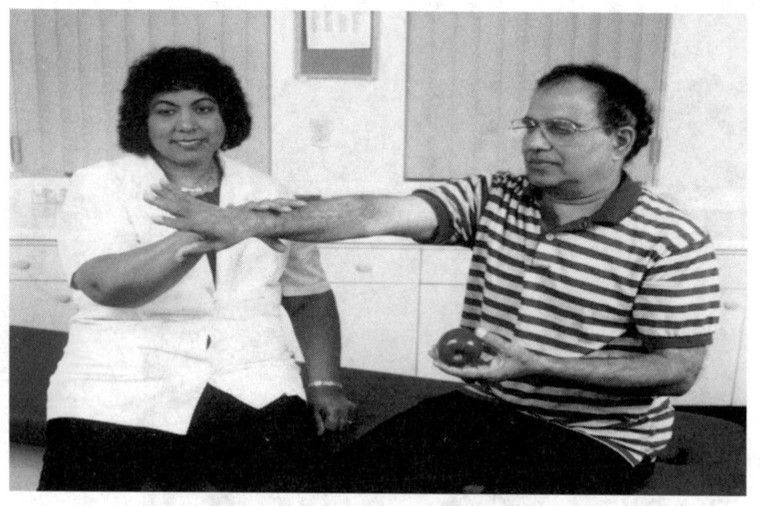

NMST IN SITTING POSITION
FIGURE 6-3

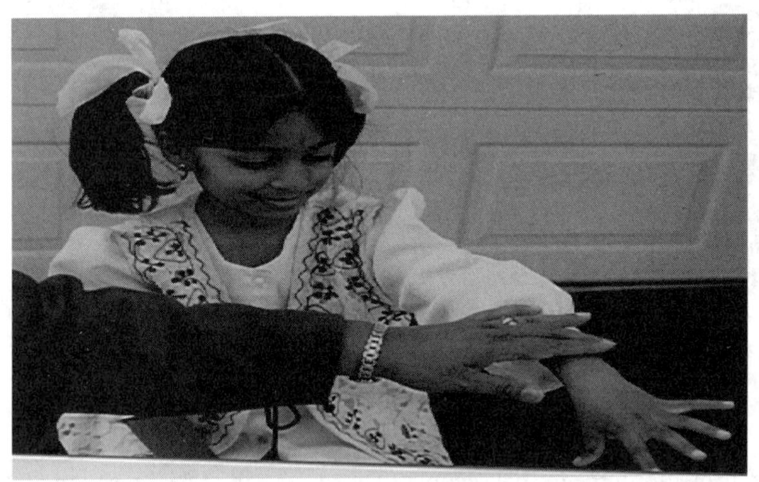

NMST IN STANDING POSITION
FIGURE 6-4

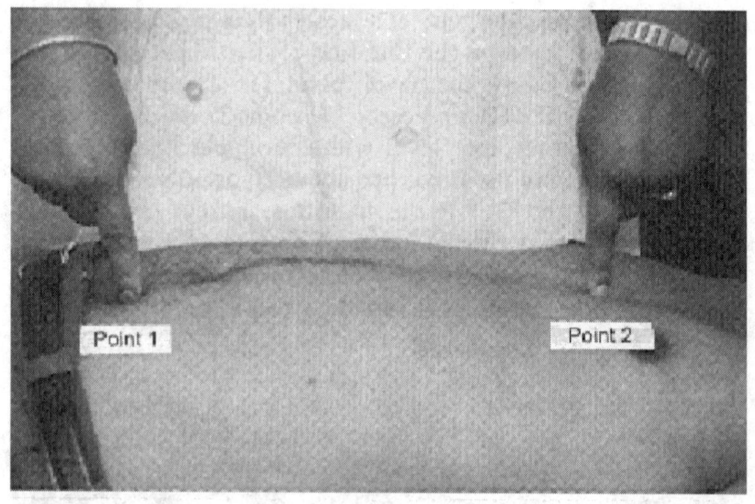

INITIAL BALANCING
FIGURE 6-5

muscle, for three to five seconds. The tester will feel a sensation of "lock" at the arm if the he is testing the arm properly and if the subject is resisting the push appropriately. If the muscle tests weak, the tester will be able to judge the difference with that small amount of pressure (5-10 lbs of pressure) he/she is applying. It may sound very easy, but much practice is needed to learn the procedure properly. If you cannot test effectively the first few times, there is no need to get frustrated. Please remember that practice makes you perfect.

Step 4: If the indicator muscle remains strong when tested without the presence of an allergen, —a sign that the subject is found to be balanced—then the tester should put the suspected allergen into the palm of the subject's resting hand. The sensory receptors, on the tips of the fingers, are extremely sensitive in recognizing allergens. When the subject's fingertips touch the allergen, the sensory receptors from the fingertips sense the charges of the allergen and relay the message to the brain. The fingertips have specialized sensory receptors that can send messages to the brain and receive the replies from the brain in a nanosecond. If the charges are compatible to the body, the indicator muscle will remain strong. If the charges are compatible, the strong PDM will go weak. This tells you that you are allergic (sensitive) to the item.

Step 5: This step is useful in balancing the patient if he/she is found to be weak on the initial testing without the presence of an allergen. You need to make the patient's test muscle strong before you can test and compare the strength of the muscle with and without the allergen. The tester places his/her fingertips of one hand at "point 1" on the midline of the subject, about one and a half inches below the navel at the conception vessel "6". The other hand is placed on conception vessel "17" (point 2), in the center of the chest on the midline, level with the nipple line. The tester massages these two points clockwise gently and simultaneously with the fingertips about 20 or 30 seconds, then repeats steps 2 and 3. If the indicator muscle tests strong, continue on to step 4. If the indicator muscle tests weak again, repeat this procedure several times. It is very unlikely that any person will remain weak after repeating this procedure two to three times.

Point 1:

Name of the point: **Sea of Energy**

Location: One and a half inches below the navel, on the midline. This is where the energy of the body is stored in abundance. When the body senses any danger around its energy field or when the body experiences energy blockages, the energy supply is cut short and stored here. If you massage clockwise on this energy reservoir point, the energy will flow out of the storage towards the energy channels and make the weak area strong again.

Point 2:

Name of the point: **Dominating Energy**

Location: In the center of the chest on the midline of the body, level with the fourth intercostal space. This is the energy dispenser unit. This is the point that controls and regulates the energy circulation in the body. When the energy rises from the *Sea of Energy*, it flows straight to the *Dominating Energy* point. From here, the energy is dispersed to different meridians, organs, tissues and cells as needed to help with the energy for body functions. It does this by forcing energy circulation from inside out. During this forced energy circulation, the blockages are pushed out of the body, bringing the body to reach a balanced state.

OVAL RING OR 'O' RING TEST

The NMST can be done in various ways. Oval ring test is another form of performing NMST. "O" ring can be used in self-testing, and this requires only one person to perform the test. This can also be used to test a subject if the subject is physically very strong with a strong arm and the tester is a physically weak person. In that case, you need two people as in standard NMST.

Step 1: The tester makes an "O" shape by opposing the little finger and thumb on the same hand. Then, with the index finger of the other hand, he/she tries to separate the "O" ring against pressure. If the ring separates easily, you need to use the balancing techniques as described in step 5 of the NMST.

Step 2: If the "O" ring remains inseparable and strong, hold the allergen in the other hand, by the fingertips, and perform step 1 again. If the "O" ring separates easily, the person is allergic to the substance he/she is touching. If the "O" ring remains strong, the substance is not an allergen.

The finger-on-finger test (Figure 6-7) is another way to test yourself. The strength of the interphalangeal muscles of two fingers of one hand is used here to test and compare the strength without and with holding an allergen. The middle finger is pushed down, using the index finger of the same hand, or vice versa, in the absence and presence of the allergen in the other hand. This also needs much practice to become good at testing.

Step 1: The tester places the pad of the index finger at the back of the middle finger of the same hand. The middle finger is pushed down, using the index finger of the same hand. If the middle finger could resist the push by the index finger, then the person is balanced. If the person is not balanced, please balance using the same step-5 from standard NMST. If the person is balanced, go to the next step.

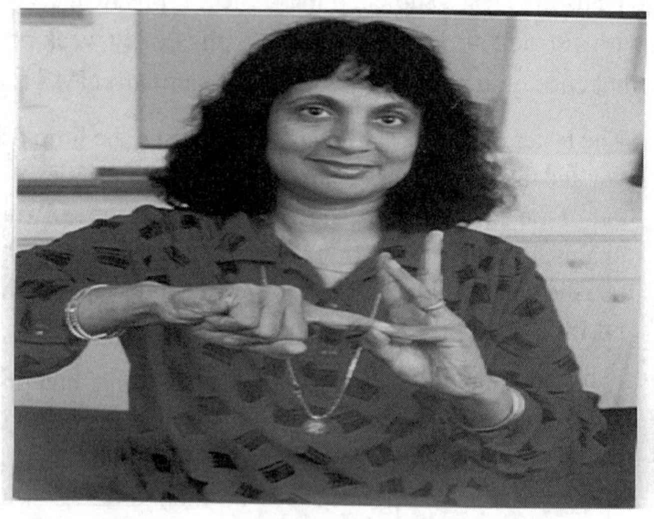

NMST WITH "O" RING TEST
FIGURE 6-6

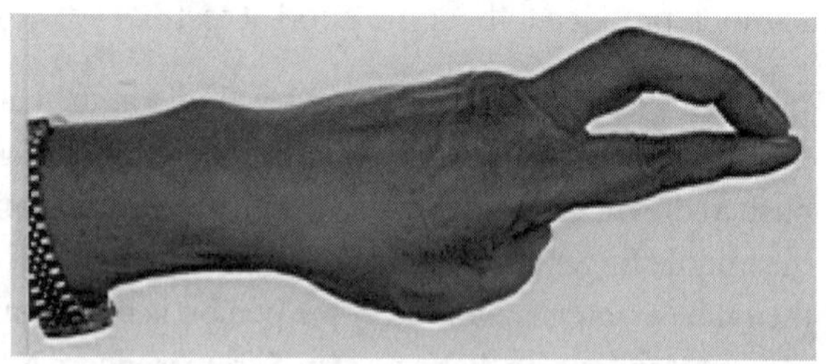

FINGER ON FINGER TEST
FIGURE 6-7

Step-2: The tester holds the allergen in one hand. Then he/she places the pad of the index finger at the back of the middle finger of the same hand again. The middle finger is pushed down, using the index finger of the same hand. The item you are holding is an allergen if the middle finger goes down easily while pushing with the index finger in the presence of the item.

NMST is one of the most reliable methods of allergy testing, and it is fairly easy to learn and practice in everyday life.

After considerable practice, some people are able to test themselves very efficiently using these methods. In order to have freedom to live in this chemically polluted world, it is very important for allergic people to learn some form of self-testing technique that enables them to screen out possible allergens before contact. This will help them prevent allergic reactions. After receiving the NAET desensitization and 100 percent clearance on NAET Classic groups (about 55 to 60 groups of allergens) from an NAET practitioner, you will be able to live normally anywhere in the world, provided you learn to self-test every item you come in contact with in the future. Hundreds of new allergens are thrown into the world daily by non-allergic people who do not understand the predicament of the allergic population. If you want to live in this world looking and feeling normal among normal people, side by side with the allergens, you need to learn how to test on your own. It is not practical for every allergic person to get treated for thousands of allergens from his/her surroundings or go to an NAET specialist every day for the rest of his/her life. You will not be free from allergies until you learn to test accurately. It takes many hours (months in some cases) of practice. But do not get discouraged. I have given enough information on testing methods here. You need to spend time and practice until you reach perfection.

A Tip to Master Self-Testing

Step-1: Find two items, or two groups of items (collect a few samples of allergens which are already tested and determined for their allergic status by another person or your NAET sp.) Then collect another group that you are not allergic to. Let's assume that you are allergic to the apple group and not allergic to the banana group in the following list.

TABLE 6-1

Group A	Group B
(Non-allergic)Apple	(Allergic)Banana
Apple	Banana
Book	Peanut
Polyester	pen
Plastc bag	Orange
The car key	Computer key board
Milk	Coffee
Cucumber	Chicken
Corn	Green pepper
Potato	Potato
Cotton	Jello-pudding

Step-2: Hold the samples from apple group one at a time in one hand and test with the other hand, using either "O" ring testing or finger on finger testing. The ring easily breaks in the case of "O" ring testing or the interphalangeal muscle weakens easily if you are using finger-on-finger testing. The same way, test each item from the banana group one by one. The "O" ring remains strong and the middle finger will not be pushed down by the index finger when you test the items from the non-allergic group.

Rub your hands together or wash your hands between touching different samples for testing.

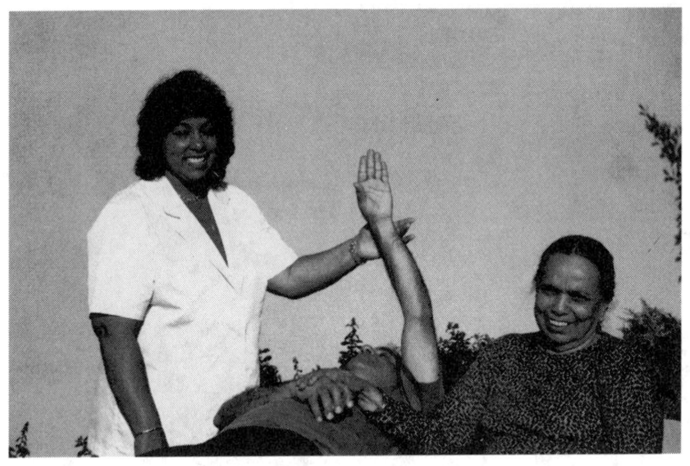

SURROGATE TESTING
FIGURE 6-8

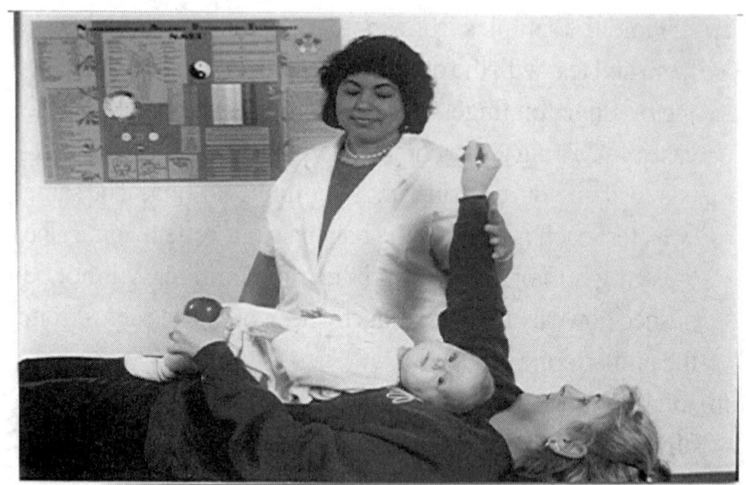

TESTING AN INFANT
FIGURE 6-9

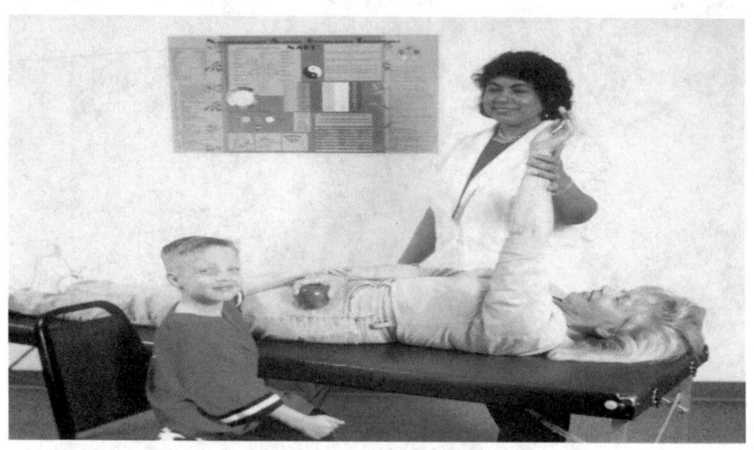

TESTING A TODDLER
FIGURE 6-10

Step-3: When you test the allergic items, if the muscle doesn't go weak, make it happen intentionally for the first few times. Now, hold the items from the non-allergic group and do the same test. This time, the ring doesn't break. Practice this procedure for awhile. Rub your hands together for 30 seconds between changing the test samples to interrupt the energy at the fingertips of the previous sample. Practice this every day until your subconscious mind is able to recognize the strength of the allergen just by touching it with your fingertips. When you master this procedure, you can test anything around you.

Surrogate Testing

This method can be very useful to test and determine the allergies of an infant, a child, an invalid or disabled person, an unconscious person, an extremely strong, or weak person, because they do not have conclusive muscle strength to perform an allergy test. You can also use this method to test an animal.

The surrogate's muscle is tested by the tester. It is important to remember to maintain skin-to-skin contact between the surrogate and the subject during the testing or desensitization procedure. If you do not maintain the skin-to-skin contact, then the surrogate will receive the results of the testing or treatment.

NAET treatments can be administered through the surrogate very effectively without causing any interference to the surrogate's energy. The testing or treatment does not affect the surrogate as long as the subject maintains uninterrupted skin-to-skin contact with him/her.

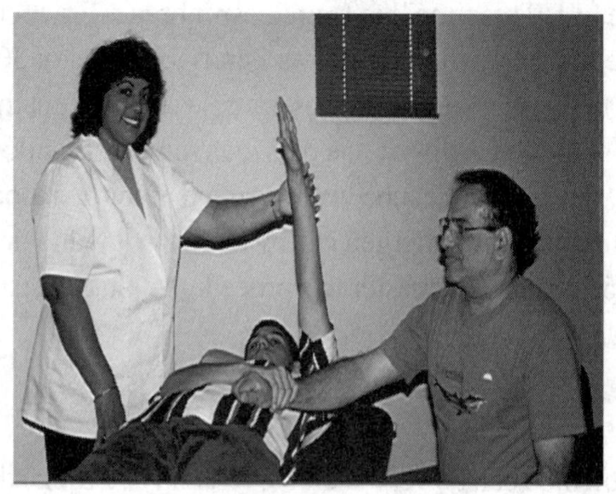

TESTING PERSON TO PERSON ALLERGY
FIGURE 6-11

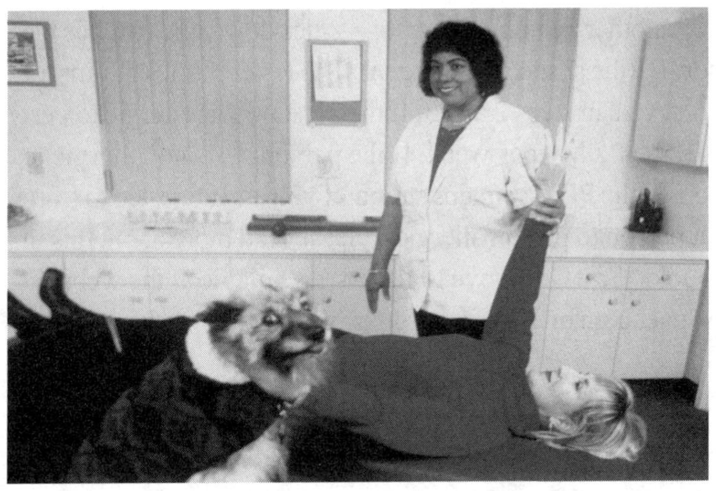

TESTING AN ANIMAL
FIGURE 6-12

You can test an allergy to anything around you using NMST. You can test your allergy to your children, spouse, friends, and other family members using this method. When you test for allergies to another person, the person-A lies down and touches the person-B (the suspected allergen). The tester pushes the arm of person-A as in steps 2 and 3. If the person-A is allergic to person-B, the PDM goes weak. If the person-A is not allergic to person-B, the PDM remains strong. If you are interested to learn about person to person allergies, please read more about this in my book, "Say Good-bye to Illness," available at the website: www.naet.com or at various bookstores in the country.

7

Acupuncture Meridians: The Pathological Symptoms

The human body is made up of bones, flesh, nerves and blood vessels, which can only function in the presence of vital energy. Like electricity, vital energy is not visible to the human eye.

No one knows how or why the vital energy gets into the body or how, when or where it goes when it leaves. It is true, however, that without it, none of the body functions can take place. When the human body is alive, vital energy flows freely through the energy pathways. Uninterrupted circulation of the vital energy flowing through the energy pathways keeps the person alive. This circulation of energy makes all the body functions possible. The circulation of the vital energy circulation makes the blood travel through the blood vessels, helping to distribute appropriate nutrients to various parts of the body for its growth, development, functions, and for repair of wear and tear.

NAET has its origin in Oriental medicine. But if one explores all the Oriental medical books, acupuncture textbooks, one may not find the NAET interpretation or evaluation about health problems that I write in my books anywhere else, because NAET is my sole development after observing my own reactions, (and my family's and patients') over the past two decades. Information about acupuncture meridians are kept to a minimum, enough to educate the reader about some of their traditional functions and possible dysfunctions in the presence of energy disturbances. Some of this information is also available in acupuncture textbooks that one may find in libraries. One needs to have some understanding about NAET evaluation of allergies and allergy-related disorders using Oriental medical knowledge to understand NAET. If anyone wishes to learn more about acupuncture meridians and mind-body connections in detail, please read Chapter 10 in my book, "Say Good-bye to Illness."

NAET utilizes a variety of standard medical procedures to diagnose allergies and then to treat allergies and allergy-related health conditions. These include: standard medical diagnostic procedures and standard allergy testing procedures (read Chapter 4) and an electro-dermal computerized allergy testing machine to detect allergies. After detecting allergies, NAET uses standard, chiropractic and acupuncture/acupressure treatments to eliminate allergies. Various studies have proven that NAET is capable of erasing the previously encoded incorrect message about an allergen and replacing it with a harmless or useful message by reprogramming the brain. This is accomplished by bringing the body into a state of "homeostasis" using other NAET energy balancing techniques.

Oriental medical theory explains the same thing from a different perspective. In Oriental medicine, the Yin-Yang state represents the perfect balance of energies (the state of homeostasis) in one's body. Any interference in the energy flow or an energy disturbance can cause an imbalance in the Yin-Yang state and an imbalance in "Homeostasis." Any substance that is capable of creating an energy disturbance in one's body is called an allergen. The result of this energy disturbance is called an allergy by my definition.

According to the NAET theory, when a substance is brought into the electromagnetic field of a person, an attraction or repulsion takes place between the energy of the person and the substance.

ATTRACTION

If two energies are attracted to each other, both energies are beneficial to each other. The living person can benefit from the association of the other substance. The energy of the substance will combine with the person and enhance the functional ability of the person many fold. For example: After taking an antibiotic, the bacterial infection is diminished in a few hours. Here the energy of the antibiotic joins forces with the energy of the body and helps to eliminate the bacteria. Another example is taking vitamin supplements and the gaining of energy and vitality.

REPULSION

If two energies are repelling each other, they are not good for each other. The living person can experience the repulsion of his/her energy from the other one as some discomfort in the body. The energy of the person will cause energy blockages in his/her energy meridians to prevent the invasion of the adverse energy into the person's energy field. For example: After taking an antibiotic, some people might react negatively because they are allergic to it and break out in a rash all over the body causing fever, excessive perspiration, light-headedness, etc. Another example is taking vitamin supplements one night and waking up with multiple joint pains and general body-ache next morning. If repulsion takes place between two energies, then the substance that is capable of producing the repulsion in a living person is called an allergen. When the allergen produces a repulsion of energy in the electromagnetic field, certain energy disturbance takes place in the body. The energy disturbance caused from the repulsion of the substance is capable of producing various unpleasant or adverse reactions in the body. These reactions are called "allergic reactions."

IMMUNOGLOBULINS

In certain instances, the body also produces many defensive forces like "Histamine, immunoglobulins, etc." to help the body to overcome the unpleasant reactions from the interaction with the allergen. Most common immunoglobulin produced during these reactions is called IgE (immunoglobulinE). These reactions are called IgE-mediated reactions. During certain reactions, specific immunoglobulins are not produced. These are called non-IgE mediated reactions. Different types of immunoglobulins are produced during allergic reactions.

An allergy means an altered reactivity. This altered reactivity can happen between two people; between one person and a nonliving substance; between one person and many nonliving substances; between one person and a living person plus one or more nonliving substances, etc.

These reactions and aftereffects can be measured using various standard medical diagnostic tests. Energy medicine has also developed various devices to measure the reactions. Oriental medicine has used *"I Ching"* almost for the same purpose since 3,322 BC. Another simple way to test one's body is through simple,

NMST, a variation of *I Ching*. It is an easy procedure to evaluate the daily progress of the patient.

Study of the acupuncture meridians is necessary to understand NAET and how it works. If one learns to identify the abnormal symptoms connected with the acupuncture meridians, detection of allergens will be easier. The pathological functions of the twelve major acupuncture meridians (energy disturbance) are given below.

The Lung Meridian (LU)

Energy disturbance in the lung meridian affecting physical and physiological levels can give rise to the following symptoms:

Afternoon fever, asthma between 3-5 a.m., atopic dermatitis, bronchitis, bronchiectasis, burning in the eyes, burning in the nostrils, cardiac asthma, chest congestion, cough, coughing up blood, cradle cap, dry mouth, dry throat, dry skin, emaciated look, emphysema, profuse perspiration, morning fatigue, fever with chills, frequent flu-like symptoms, headache between eyes, general body ache with burning sensation, generalized hives, hair loss, hair thinning, hay-fever, infantile eczema, infection in the respiratory tract, itching of the nostrils, itching of the body, itching of the scalp, lack of perspiration, lack of desire to talk, laryngitis, low voice, night sweats, mucus in the throat, nasal congestion, nose bleed, pain in the chest and intercostal muscles, between third and fourth thoracic vertebrae, in the first interphalangeal joint, in the upper first and second cuspids (tooth), in the thumb, in the upper back, in the eyes, and in the upper arms; pleurisy, pharyngitis, pneumonia, poor growth of nails and hair, postnasal drip, red cheeks, red eyes, restlessness between 3 to 5 a.m., runny nose with clear discharge, thin or thick white discharge in case of viral infection, thick yellow discharge in case of bacterial infection, tonsillitis, scaly and rough skin, skin rashes, skin tags, moles, sinus infections, sinus headaches, sneezing, sore throat, stuffy nose, swollen throat, swollen cervical glands, tenosynovitis, throat irritation, warts, and inability to sleep after 3 am.

Energy disturbance in the lung meridian affecting the cellular level may cause the following:

Cellular level blockage of lung meridian often expresses grief or sadness. When one fails to cry, when one feels deep sorrow, sadness will settle in the lungs and eventually cause various lung disorders. Other symptoms of cellular level imbalance: Apologizing, comparing self with others, contempt, dejection, depression, despair, false pride, hopelessness, intolerance, likes to humiliate others, loneliness, low self-esteem, meanness, melancholy, over sympathy, over demanding, prejudice, seeking others' approval in doing things, self pity, highly sensitive emotionally, and weeping frequently without much reason.

Essential nutrients to strengthen the lung meridian:

Clear water, proteins, vitamin C, bioflavonoid, cinnamon, onions, garlic, B-vitamins (especially B_2), citrus fruits, green peppers, black peppers and brown rice. If one is allergic to any of these essential nutrients, it can act as a trigger to asthma or any other respiratory problem.

The Large Intestine Meridian (LI)

Energy disturbance in the large intestine meridian affecting physical and physiological levels can give rise to the following symptoms:

Abdominal pain, acne on the face especially sides of the mouth and nose, asthma after 5 a.m., asthma, arthritis of the shoulder joint, arthritis of the knee joint, arthritis of the index finger, arthritis of the wrist joint, arthritis of the lateral part of the elbow and hip, bad breath, blisters in the lower gum, bursitis, dermatitis, dry mouth and thirst, eczema, fatigue, feeling better after a bowel movement, or feeling tired after a bowel movement, flatulence, inflammation of lower gum, intestinal colic, itching of the body, loose stools or constipation, lower backache, headaches, muscle spasms and pain of lateral thigh and knee, motor impairment of the fingers, pain in the knee, pain in the shoulder and shoulder blade, back of the neck, pain and swelling of the index finger, pain in the lateral aspect of the leg below the knee joint, pain in the heel, sciatic pain, swollen cervical glands, shortness of breath, skin rashes, skin tags, sinusitis, tenosynovitis, tennis elbow, toothache, warts on the skin.

Energy disturbance in the large intestine meridian affecting the cellular level can cause the following:

Guilt, constipation of the mind, bad dreams, dwelling on past memory, crying spells, defensiveness, inability to recall dreams, nightmares, nostalgia, rolling restlessly in sleep, sadness, seeking sympathy, talking in the sleep and weeping.

Essential nutrients to strengthen the large intestine meridian:

Vitamins A, D, E, C, B, especially B_1, wheat, wheat bran, oat bran, yoghurt, and roughage. If one is allergic to any of these essential nutrients, it can act as a trigger to asthma or any other respiratory problem.

The Stomach Meridian (ST)

Energy disturbance in the stomach meridian affecting physical and physiological levels can give rise to the following symptoms:

Abdominal distention, acid reflux disorders, acne on the face and neck, ADD, ADHD, anorexia, asthma accompanied by nausea or vomiting, autism, bad breath, black and blue marks on the leg below the knee, bipolar disorders, blemishes, bulimia, chest muscle pain, coated tongue, coldness in the lower limbs, cold sores in the mouth, delirium, depression, dry nostrils, dyslexia, facial paralysis, fever blisters, fibromyalgia, flushed face, frontal headache, heat boils (painful, reddish, acne) in the upper front of the body, herpes, hiatal hernia, high fever, learning disability, insomnia due to nervousness, itching on the skin below the knee, migraine headaches, manic depressive disorders, nasal polyps, nausea, nosebleed, pain on the upper jaws, pain in the mid-back, pain in the eye, persistent hunger, red rashes, seizures, sensitivity to cold, shortness of breath, sore throat, sore tongue, sores on the gums, stomach ache, sweating, swelling on the neck, temporomandibular joint problem, unable to relax the mind or stop thinking, upper gum diseases and vomiting.

Energy disturbance in the stomach meridian affecting the cellular level can cause the following:

Disgust, bitterness, aggressive behaviors, attention deficit disorders, butterfly sensation in the stomach, constant thinking, depression, deprivation, despair, disappointment, egotism, emptiness, greed, hyperactivity, manic disorder, mental fog, mental confusion, nervousness, nostalgia, obsession, paranoia, poor concentration, poor memory, restlessness and schizophrenia.

Essential nutrients to strengthen the stomach meridian:

B complex especially B_{12}, B_6, B_3 and folic acid.

The Spleen Meridian (SP)

Energy disturbance in the spleen meridian affecting physical and physiological levels can give rise to the following symptoms:

Abnormal taste, abnormal smell, abnormal uterine bleeding, absence of menstruation, asthma, alzheimer's disease, autism, bleeding under the skin, bleeding from the mucous membrane, bruises under the skin, bitter taste in the mouth, cold sores on the lips, carpal tunnel syndrome, coldness of the legs, chronic gastro-enteritis, cramps after the first day of menses, depression, diabetes, dizzy spells, dreams that make you tired, emaciated muscles, failing memory, fatigue in general, fatigued limbs, fatigue of the mind, feverishness, fibromyalgia, fluttering of the eyelids, generalized edema, hard lumps in the abdomen, hemophilia, hemorrhoids, hyperglycemia, hypoglycemia, hypertension, inability to make decisions, incontinence of urine, or stool, indigestion, infertility, insomnia usually unable to fall asleep, intractable pain anywhere in the body, intuitive and prophetic behaviors, irregular periods, lack of enthusiasm, lack of interest in anything, lethargy, light headedness, loose stools, nausea, obesity, pain in the great toes, pain and stiffness of the fingers, pallor, pedal edema, prolapse of the uterus, poor memory, prolapse of the bladder, purpura, reduced appetite, sand-like feeling in the eyes, scanty menstrual flow, small, frequent, pencil-like thin stools with undigested food particles, sensation of heaviness in the head, sensation of heaviness in the body, shortness of breath, sleep during the day, sluggishness, slowing of the mind, swollen eyelids, swollen lips, swellings or pain with swelling of the toes and feet, fingers and hands, swelling anywhere in the body, stiffness of the tongue, sugar craving, tingling or abnormal sensation in the tip of the fingers and palms, varicose veins, vomiting, and watery eyes.

Energy disturbance in the spleen meridian affecting the cellular level can cause the following:

Worry, concern, anxiety, does not like crowds, easily hurt, gives more importance to self, hopelessness, irritable, keeps feelings inside, lack of confidence, likes loneliness, likes to take revenge, likes to be praised, likes to get constant encouragement — otherwise falls apart, lives through others, low self esteem, obsessive compulsive behavior, over sympathetic to others, restrained, shy, talks to self, timid, and unable to make decisions.

Essential nutrients to strengthen the spleen meridian:

Vitamin A, vitamin C, calcium, chromium, protein and sugar. If one is allergic to any of these essential nutrients, it can act as a trigger to asthma or any other respiratory problem.

The Heart Meridian (HT)

Energy disturbance in the heart meridian affecting physical and physiological levels can give rise to the following symptoms:

Angina-like pains, chest pains, discomfort when reclining, dizziness, dry throat, excessive perspiration, feverishness, headache, heart palpitation, heaviness in the chest, hot palms and soles, insomnia—unable to fall asleep when awakened in the middle of sleep, irritability, mental disorders, nervousness, pain in the eye, pain along the left arm, pain along the scapula, pain and fullness in the chest, poor circulation, shortness of breath, and shoulder pains.

Energy disturbance in the heart meridian affecting the cellular level can cause the following:

Joy, or lack of joy, self-confidence, compassion and love are the emotions of the heart. But when the energy is blocked, one may experience the following: abusive nature, anger, aggression, bad manners, lack of love and compassion, compulsive behaviors, does not trust anyone, does not like to make friends, easily upset, excessive laughing or crying, guilt, hostility, insecurity, lack of emotions, overexcitement, sadness, and type A personality.

Essential nutrients to strengthen the heart meridian:

Calcium, vitamin C, vitamin E, fatty acids, selenium, potassium, sodium, iron, and B complex.

The Small Intestine Meridian (SI)

Energy disturbance in the small intestine meridian affecting physical and physiological levels can give rise to the following symptoms:

Abdominal pain, abdominal fullness, acne on the upper back, bad breath, bitter taste in the mouth, constipation, diarrhea, distention of lower abdomen, dry stool, frozen shoulder, knee pain, night sweats, numbness of the mouth and tongue, numbness of the back of the shoulder and arm, pain in the neck, pain radiating around the waist, shoulder pain, sore throat, stiff neck, pain along the lateral aspect of the shoulder and arm.

Energy disturbance in the small intestine meridian affecting the cellular level can cause the following:

Insecurity, absent-mindedness, becoming too involved with details, day dreaming, easily annoyed, emotional instability, feeling of abandonment, feeling shy, having a tendency to be introverted and easily hurt, irritability, excessive joy or lack of joy, lacking- confidence, over excitement, paranoia, poor concentration, sadness, sighing, sorrow, suppressing deep sorrow.

Essential nutrients to strengthen the small intestine meridian:

Vitamin B complex, vitamin D, vitamin E, acidophilus, yoghurt, fibers, fatty acids, spices, wheat germ and whole grains.

The Bladder Meridian (BL)

Energy disturbance in the bladder meridian affecting physical and physiological levels can give rise to the following symptoms:

Arthritis of the joints of little finger, bloody urine, burning urination, chills, chronic headaches at the back of the neck, disease of the eye, enuresis, fever, frequent urination, headaches especially at the back of the neck, loss of bladder control, mental disorders, muscle wasting, nasal congestion, pain and discomfort in the lower abdomen, pain in the inner canthus of the eyes, pain behind the knees, pain and stiffness of the back, pain in the fingers and toes, pain in the lateral part of the sole, pain in the lower back, pain along back of the leg and foot, pain in the lateral part of the ankle, pain along the meridian, pain in the little toe, painful urination, retention of urine, sciatic neuralgia, shortness of breath on exertion, spasm behind the knee, spasms along the posterior part of the thigh and leg, spasms of the calf muscles, stiff neck, weakness in the rectum and rectal muscle.

Energy disturbance in the bladder meridian affecting the cellular level can cause the following:

Fright, fear, sadness, disturbing and impure thoughts, annoyed, fearful, unhappy, frustrated, highly irritable, impatient, inefficient, insecure, reluctant and restless.

Essential nutrients to strengthen the bladder meridian:

Vitamin C, A, E, B complex, especially B_1, calcium, amino acids and trace minerals. If one is allergic to any of these essential nutrients, it can act as a trigger to asthma or any other respiratory problem.

The Kidney Meridian (KI)

Energy disturbance in the kidney meridian affecting physical and physiological levels can give rise to the following symptoms:

Bags under the eyes, blurred vision, burning or painful urination, chronic diarrhea, coldness in the back, cold feet, crave salt, dark circles under the eyes, dryness of the mouth, excessive sleeping, excessive salivation, excessive thirst, facial edema, fatigue, fever with chills, frequent urination, impotence, irritability, light headedness, lower backache, motor impairment, muscular atrophy of the foot, nagging mild asthma, nausea, pain in the sole of the foot, pain in the posterior aspect of the leg or thigh, pain in the ears, poor memory, poor concentration, poor appetite, puffy eyes, ringing in the ears, sore throat, shortness of breath on exertion, spasms of the ankle and feet, swelling in the legs, swollen ankles and vertigo.

Energy disturbance in the kidney meridian affecting the cellular level can cause the following:

Fear, terror, caution, confused, indecision, seeks attention, unable to express feelings.

Essential nutrients to strengthen the kidney meridian:

Vitamins A, E, B, essential fatty acids, amino acids, sodium chloride, trace minerals, calcium and iron. If one is allergic to any of these essential nutrients, it can act as a trigger to asthma or any other respiratory problem.

The Pericardium Meridian (PC)

Energy disturbance in the pericardium meridian affecting physical and physiological levels can give rise to the following symptoms:

Chest pain, cardiac asthma, contracture of the arm or elbow, excessive appetite, fainting spells, flushed face, frozen shoulder, fullness in the chest, heaviness in the chest, hot palms and soles, impaired speech, irritability, nausea, nervousness, pain in the anterior part of the thigh, pain in the eyes, pain in the medial part of the knee, palpitation, restricting movements, sensation of hot or cold, slurred speech, spasms of the elbow, arm and motor impairment of the tongue.

Energy disturbance in the pericardium meridian affecting the cellular level can cause the following:

Shock, hurt, extreme joy, fear of heights, heaviness in the head, heaviness in the chest due to emotional overload, imbalance in sexual energy like never having enough sex, jealousy, light sleep with dreams, manic disorders, in some cases no desire for sex, over- excitement, regret, sexual tension, stubbornness and various phobias.

Essential nutrients to strengthen the pericardium meridian:

Vitamin E, vitamin C, chromium, and trace minerals.

The Triple Warmer Meridian (TW)

Energy disturbance in the triple warmer meridian affecting physical and physiological levels can give rise to the following symptoms:

Abdominal pain, always feels hungry even after eating a full meal, constipation, deafness, distention, dysuria, edema, enuresis, excessive thirst, excessive hunger, fever in the late evening, frequent urination, hardness and fullness in the lower abdomen, indigestion, pain in the medial part of the knee, pain in the shoulder and upper arm, pain behind the ear, pain in the cheek and jaw, redness in the eye, shoulder pain, swelling and pain in the throat and vertigo.

Energy disturbance in the triple warmer meridian affecting the cellular level can cause the following:

Depression, deprivation, despair, emptiness, excessive emotion, grief, hopelessness and phobias.

Essential nutrients to strengthen the triple warmer meridian:

Iodine, trace minerals, vitamin C, calcium, fluoride and water.

The Gall Bladder Meridian (GB)

Energy disturbance in the gall bladder meridian affecting physical and physiological levels can give rise to the following symptoms:

A heavy sensation in the right upper part of the abdomen, abdominal bloating, alternating fever and chills, ashen complexion, bitter taste in the mouth, burping after meals, chills, deafness, dizziness, fever, headaches on the sides of the head, heartburn after fatty foods, hyperacidity, moving arthritis, pain in the jaw, nausea with fried foods, pain in the eye, pain in the hip, pain and cramps along the anterolateral wall, poor digestion of fats, sciatic neuralgia, shortness of breath, sighing, stroke-like condition, swelling in the submaxillary region, tremors, twitching, vision disturbances, vomiting and yellowish complexion.

Energy disturbance in the gall bladder meridian affecting the cellular level can cause the following:

Gall bladder is associated with control issues, rage, aggression, complaining all the time, fearful, finding faults with others and unhappiness.

Essential nutrients to strengthen the gall bladder meridian:

Vitamin A, apples, lemon, calcium, linoleic acids and oleic acids (for example, pine nuts, olive oil). If one is allergic to any of these essential nutrients, it can act as a trigger to asthma or any other respiratory problem.

The Liver Meridian (LV)

Energy disturbance in the liver meridian affecting physical and physiological levels can give rise to the following symptoms:

Abdominal pain, blurred vision, dark urine, dizziness, enuresis, excessive bright colored bleeding during menses, feeling of some obstruction in the throat, fever, hard lumps in the upper abdomen, headache at the top of the head, hernia, hemiplegia, irregular menses, jaundice, loose stools, pain in the intercostal region, pain in the breasts, pain in the lower abdomen, paraplegia, PMS, reproductive organ disturbances, retention of urine, seizures, shortness of breath after getting exposed to chemicals, spasms in the extremities, stroke-like condition, tinnitus, vertigo, and vomiting.

Energy disturbance in the liver meridian affecting the cellular level can cause the following:

Anger, irritability, aggression, assertion, rage, shouting, talking loud and type A personality.

Essential nutrients to strengthen the liver meridian:

Beets, green vegetables, vitamin A, trace minerals and unsaturated fatty acids.

The Governing Vessel Meridian (GV)

Energy disturbance in the governing vessel meridian affecting physical, physiological and psychological levels can give rise to the following symptoms:

This channel supplies the brain and spinal region and intersects the liver channel at the vertex. Obstruction of its Chi may result in symptoms such as stiffness and pain along the spinal column. Deficient Chi in the channel may produce a heavy sensation in the head, vertigo and shaking. Energy blockages in this meridian (which passes through the brain) may be responsible for certain mental disorders. Febrile diseases are commonly associated with the governing vessel channel and because one branch of the channel ascends through the abdomen, when the channel is unbalanced, its Chi rushes upward toward the heart. Symptoms such as colic, constipation, enuresis, hemorrhoids and functional infertility may result.

The Conception Vessel Meridian (CV, REN)

Energy disturbance in the conception vessel meridian affecting physical, physiological and psychological levels can give rise to the following symptoms:

The conception vessel channel is the confluence of the Yin channels. Therefore, abnormality along the conception vessel channel will appear principally in pathological symptoms of the Yin channels, especially symptoms associated with the liver and kidneys. Its function is closely related with pregnancy and, therefore, has intimate links with the kidneys and uterus. If its Chi is deficient, infertility or other disorders of the urogenital system may result. Leukorrhea, irregular menstruation, colic, etc., are associated with the conception vessel channel.

Any allergen can cause blockage in one or more meridians at the same time. If it is causing blockages in only one meridian, the patient may demonstrate symptoms related to that particular meridian. The intensity of the symptoms will depend on the severity of the blockage. The patient may suffer from one symptom, many symptoms or all the symptoms of this meridian. Sometimes, a patient can have many meridians blocked at the same time. In such cases, the patient may demonstrate a variety of symptoms, one symptom from each meridian or many symptoms from certain meridians and one or two from other meridians. Some patients with blockage in one meridian can demonstrate just one symptom from the list, but may be with great intensity.

Some people, even though they have disturbances in all meridians, may not show any symptoms. Such patients might have a better immune system than others. Variations with all these possibilities make diagnosis difficult in some cases.

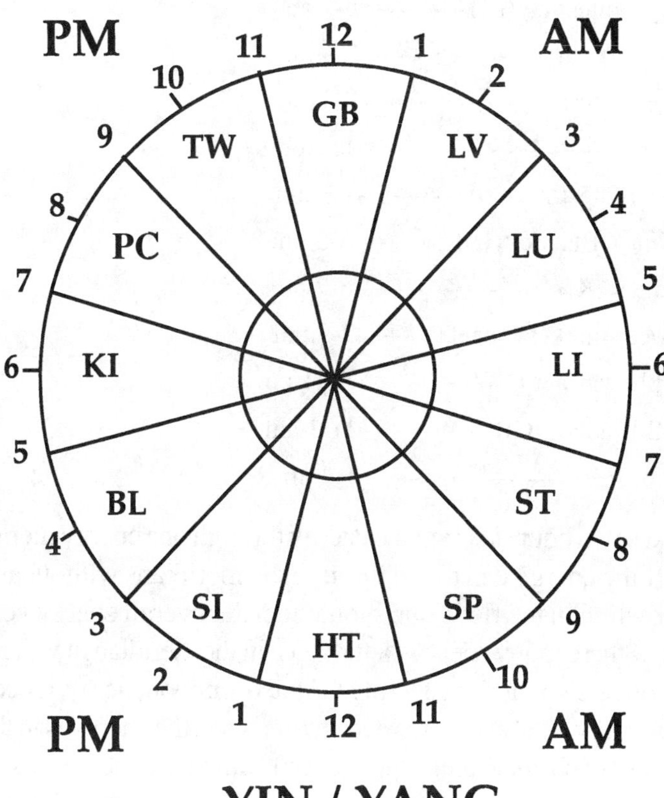

FIGURE 7-1
ORGAN-MERIDIAN ASSOCIATION
CLOCK

Names of the Meridians and Corresponding Hours

Lung (Lu) ---------------------3-5 am

Large Intestine (LI) ---------- 5-7 am

Stomach (St) ----------------- 7-9 am

Spleen (Sp) ------------------- 9-11am

Heart -------------------------- 11-1pm

Small Intestine - (SI) ----------1-3 pm

Urinary Bladder (UB) -------- 3-5 pm

Kidney (Ki) ------------------- 5-7 pm

Pericardium (PC or CI) ----- -7-9 pm

Triple warmer (TW) -----------9-11 pm

Gall Bladder (GB) ----------- 11-1 am

Liver (Lv) ---------------------1-3 am

It takes two hours to circulate energy through one energy meridian. If the energy can travel through the meridians without any obstruction in the flow, one should feel the overall energy very high. If there is any energy disturbance in the meridian, it will reflect on one's health by feeling fatigued or poor energy. Check your energy level every two even hours when the energy is in the center of each meridian: Check at 6:00 am to find out the status of Large Intestine meridian, etc. (5-7 am is the meridian time for LI). After you find your weak time find the corresponding meridian (s) from the list below. Then go to the respective meridian in this Chapter (Also you will find detailed information about these acupuncture meridians in *Say Good-bye to Illness in* Chapter 10) to find out more about your health. Then go to Chapter 9 to learn the self-balancing techniques. Do it once or twice a day for a few weeks. No matter what condition you are in, your energy will get better.

8

Living with Asthma

We have seen how asthma can interfere with people's lives, how it can complicate one's existence and take the pleasure out of living.

If you take time to look around, you will be amazed to find that most people with asthma live the lives of prisoners: No freedom to eat; no freedom to drink; no freedom to breathe; no freedom to sleep; no freedom to wear the clothes they like to; no freedom to use makeup; no freedom to use certain chemicals; no freedom to go to certain places; no freedom to be with people they like to be with; because they have to live within a certain area; they have to eat certain foods; they have to abstain from their favorite food; they have to live near hospitals; they have to carry a nebulizer whereever they go; they have to carry oxygen when they travel; they have to be taking medication round the clock; if they miss one medication, they will have to pay the price. In fact, a prisoner has more freedom to do things in his/her life than an asthmatic victim. An asthmatic person is so fearful because he/she does not have a clue when the big attack will put him/her right back in the intensive care unit!

Trapped for life?

Is there a way out?

Do you have to live rest of your life in fear like this?

No, certainly not. You do not have to be a prisoner of your own disease. You can have freedom to do anything you want to and freedom to live again if you carefully read this Chapter and follow the suggestions given in this Chapter.

Also, please read Chapter 6. Using the testing methods described in Chapter 6, you can learn to test your allergies to the products that you come in contact with before you use them in your everyday life. Then, avoid the items that are not good for your body. Early on, if there are certain items that you cannot avoid, get a few NAET treatments to lessen your sensitivity. After successfully clearing the allergy to the allergens, you will be able to use them without any further adverse reaction which will put you on the road to freedom from your asthma.

If you learn the testing procedures and practice at home, it won't be long before you find out that most of your health problems (or your loved one's) have their roots in your daily diets, or clothes, even in the vitamins you were using which you thought were helping you to live healthy and well. Many of your health problems could be caused by the items in your daily life.

How Surprised You Will Be When You Discover:

Your 23-year suffering from asthma was due to an allergy to eggs and aggravated by egg, as you prepared muffins, pancakes, and waffles for guests at your bed and breakfast facility every morning.

An allergy to your soft, expensive feather pillow was causing your chronic sinusitis.

Your nasal congestion and chronic bronchitis were due to an allergy to beet-pulp that was fed the cows on a daily basis and excreted in their milk and assimilated by you via the three glasses of milk you drank daily hoping to reduce osteoporosis by drinking milk.

Your daily nighttime asthma was due to an allergy to the artificial sweetener used in the mouthwash you rinsed your mouth with before bedtime every night.

Waking up every night around 1:00 a.m. was due to an allergy to the detergent you used to wash your bed linen.

Soon after you bought your expensive rocking chair that gave you so much pleasure to sit on the balcony and watch the passersby, you began getting regular asthmatic attacks after a half-hour. Did you know your everyday, 5:00 p.m. asthma was caused by the widely used flame-retardant chemical PBDE (Polybrominated diphenyl ethers) in the foam cushions of the rocking chair?

Your child's chronic bronchitis was probably due to an allergy to that one glass of orange juice he drinks every morning.

Your allergy to humidity caused you to feel suffocated in the shower when you were forced to shower with the doors and windows open.

Your six-year-old son was allergic to cold (snow) and dampness that caused his asthma at the ski resort when you had to rush him to hospital.

The peanut butter in the chocolate bar triggered your asthma last night and your family had to call "911."

Pollens brought in by the Santa Ana wind and deposited in your neighborhood caused your asthma as soon as you walked to the "Deli."

When you went to the market, you passed by that beautiful girl who wore the sweet perfume and you stayed around her for awhile longer, got a few more whiffs of her perfume and in the next ten minutes the shopkeeper had to call 911, and after which you were taken to the hospital for your sudden severe asthma attack. Did you know that perfume triggered the asthma?

Every time your little daughter hugged the stuffed toy it triggered an asthma. Did you know the filling of stuffed bear was responsible for her asthma whenever she played with it?

Your child's frequent colds and sore throat were due to an allergy to the city water he drinks at school.

Your husband's two-month-old walking pneumonia was due to an allergy to the yoghurt he eats daily for lunch at work.

Awakening with asthma every morning at 4:00 a.m. was due to the gentle over-the-counter laxative you took every night?

The shocking fact is that if one evaluates carefully, everything around you is a potential allergen that can trigger an asthmatic attack at any time. If you learn how to test and find your allergies, before they trigger an asthma situation, you could prevent asthma. Now you have a way to do just that. You can test and find your allergies within the privacy of your own home, without going through expensive and extensive laboratory tests. (Caution: If you are suffering from a major asthma or asthma-related disorder, please see your doctor or appropriate specialist immediately and get evaluated first.) By avoiding the allergens in your life, you will be able to live peacefully without suffering from asthma. If you must use the products, please see a practitioner who is trained in NAET. If you take time to read this book, you will understand how to help yourself with mild to moderate asthmatic symptoms, because some self-balancing tips are given in Chapter 9. If you are a person with many allergies, with severe asthmatic symptoms, please consult a pulmonologist and an NAET specialist right away to get appropriate evaluation and a few NAET treatments before you try self-help procedures. For complicated problems, you need to see an appropriate specialist.

Everyone should be tested and treated for all NAET Basic allergen groups. NAET basic treatments include the basic essentials of life, the most commonly used food and enzymes from everyday life. By eliminating the allergies to the essential nutrients, one's overall immunity will improve, with the result that one may not suffer new allergies or asthmatic symptoms.

It will help you to learn certain rules before beginning treatments with a NAET doctor.

Instructions to the Patient Before Beginning NAET

1. Patients should be encouraged to read *Say Good-bye To Illness* before they begin the NAET treatments. Doctor should explain the treatment procedure to the patient before beginning the treatment.

2. If you have any laboratory reports from a previous doctor, please bring them with you.

3. Please do not wear any perfume, perfumed powder, strong smelling deodorant, hair spray, or after shave, eat strong smelling

herbs like raw garlic, etc., when you come to the clinic for treatments. Do not bring any little children or pets to the clinic when you come for the treatment. No one should sit or stand in the room when the doctor is testing or treating the patient. The presence of a third person or animal can negate your treatment if the third person is standing in your energy field.

4. There is no smoking allowed in (or around) the office. Please do not wear clothes that smell like smoke or paint. Other patients could react to these smells.

5. Please wash your hands before and after the treatment. Or, after the treatment, instead of washing the hands, vigorous rubbing of the hands for 30 seconds will be sufficient.

6. Do not exercise for six hours after the treatment.

7. Avoid exposure to extreme hot or cold temperature after the treatment.

8. Please take a shower before you come in for a treatment, and wear freshly washed clothes to avoid the smell of herbs, spices, perspiration, etc. from your body or clothes. This can cause irritation and reactions in other allergic patients.

9. Do not bathe or shower until six hours after the treatment.

10. Do not eat or chew gum or candy during the treatment.

11. After each NAET treatment, you are required to wait in the office for 20 minutes. Do not cross your hands or feet during the first 20 minutes after the treatment.

12. Do not read or touch other objects during the 20 minutes following the treatment because contact with other substances during this period could cause your treatment to fail.

13. Wear minimum or no jewelry when you come for a treatment. Avoid wearing large crystals or large diamonds.

14. For best results, after each treatment, the treated allergen must be avoided for 25 hours or more. The patients who follows 25-hour avoidance get the best results from NAET. During 25 hours, the body goes through natural detoxification. Often these patients do not need to go through other detoxification procedures. If you need more hours of waiting period after the treatment, your NAET specialist can check for this and inform you after each treatment. Remember to recheck with your doctor for the item you treated, after 25 hours, and at least within one week to make sure you have completed the treatment. If you did not complete the treatment, your symptoms due to the incomplete treatment may continue for a long time, sometimes for weeks.

NAET treatments follow a given order; the Basics come first.

If you are in the doctor's office with an acute reaction, your doctor (practitioner) may treat you for the allergen causing the acute reaction. That is the only time a true NAET doctor will treat out of the given order.

If your practitioner is not confident to treat your acute problem using NAET, please go to the nearest emergency room or if you are too sick to travel, please call 911 immediately.

15. To insure maximum progress with your treatments, maintain your own treatment and food diary in the NAET guide book at the section for record keeping. If you need help to record your treatments, please ask your practitioner.

16. You may need to take extra precautions while you get treated for environmental substances: (mineral mix, metals, water, leather, formaldehyde, fabric, wood, mold, mercury, newspaper,

marker ink, chemicals, flowers, perfume, etc.). Apart from staying away from the item, you may also need to wear mask, gloves, socks and shoes even to bed, full gowns, scarf, earplugs, covering your head, ear, and forehead, etc. for 25 hours following treatment.

17. Always eat before you come for the treatment. You should not take NAET with acupuncture treatments when you are hungry. If you have a long wait in your doctor's office, please bring a snack with you and eat it away from other patients just before the treatment

18. Do not eat heavy meals after the NAET treatments.

19. Drink a glass of water before the treatment. Energy moves better in a well hydrated body. Drink lots of water (4-6 glasses/day) after each NAET treatment to help flush out the toxins produced during the treatment.

20. Please do not stop any other treatment you are on: medication, therapy, chiropractic treatments, acupuncture, massages, etc. It is good for your body to have a general body massage before the NAET or 6 hours after NAET treatments. Massages can help to improve the energy flow through the energy pathways. If you are taking lots of vitamins and herbs, or any particular drug, continue them as before if you think that they are helping you. But when you get treated for the food containing a particular vitamin, herb, or substance, at certain times you may be asked to stop the vitamin, herbs, or drugs for 25 hours following that particular treatment, or to use a substitute.

21. NAET treatment will not interfere with any other treatment. In fact, if you can keep your body free of toxin accumulation (stool softeners, laxatives, to prevent constipation, and colonics or high enemas once or twice a month to eliminate the toxic

buildup), and keep your symptoms under control with whatever method you are using, NAET treatment will be a lot easier.

22. NAET for allergens are not advisable when the patient is extremely tired, worked long hours, or has worked the night shift without any rest, is extremely hungry, or has experienced an emotional trauma within the past few hours. A simple NAET balancing treatment will be better in such situations.

23. You can learn how to test your allergies at home for your daily usable items and self-treat to handle possible emergencies.

24. If you are having a difficult time to pass an allergen, your doctor can teach you to massage general balancing points every two hours while awake by just thinking about the sample.

25. For female patients: Treatments are not advisable during the first three days of the menstrual cycle.

26. Patients are advised to take a break from the treatment after completing difficult items.

Importance of Finding the Right Causative Allergen

I spent countless hours testing, determining, researching, and trying out all my NAET discoveries on hundreds of people before I began sharing them with others. I was a desperate patient myself some time ago. I was told to learn to live with my chronic health problems for the rest of my life. So I understand the pain of living with sickness and feeling trapped.

Now, we have a simple, safe, inexpensive, uncomplicated procedure to test asthma and allergies with maximum accuracy.

It is very important to find the right culprit that causes your asthma. It may be the simple tap water, bottled water, the fruits you picked from your tree, the vegetable you bought from the market, the cane sugar you added in your morning tea, the smell of brewing your morning coffee, the detergent you bought last week. Whatever may be the cause, you need to find that one major trigger to treat any acute attacks. If someone gets repeated attacks, as do chronic asthmatics, the asthma may not be caused from one allergen. It may be due to exposures from multiple allergens. In that case, a single treatment may not produce a satisfactory result. All known allergens should be eliminated one by one in a specific order, the most important one first, eventually all. In some cases, it may take months or even a couple of years before you can eliminate all known allergens. That's why we group the allergens in a specific manner when treating nonacute allergic patients or chronic asthma cases, in order to give maximum benefits in a minimum amount of time and visits. While going through the treatment phase, patients are required to continue all the supporting drugs that are necessary to keep their asthma under control.

You can test any type of allergen using NAET testing methods described in Chapter 6. I am going to list a few commonly encountered, unsuspected, allergens below. When I tell someone to test each and every item before using, most people do not understand that one could be allergic to a vast number of everyday items around them. Most people, including some practitioners, miss unsuspected, hidden allergens. These innocent looking allergens may be the cause of seemingly incurable diseases. Let us look at a case study of one of my patients:

A 42-year-old athlete bought a large case of fig bars for snacks from a store. He liked the taste and began eating many bars the first day. By the second day he came down with a common cold, chills, fever. In a few more days, the cold turned into upper respiratory infection with cough, fever, general fatigue. He lived alone, had no energy to cook or go out to eat. He had no appetite except for the fig bar. He took sick leave from work, began to sleep most of the day without having any energy or motivation to do any chores.

His continuous cough irritated him and made him more tired. Soon he developed high fever along with the upper respiratory infection. Finally he went to see his internist. His upper respiratory infection turned into pneumonia. His doctor prescribed antibiotics for ten days. His symptoms persisted in spite of antibiotics and inhalers. After seven days of antibiotics, his problems continued to get worse. At that time, one of his friends brought him to my office for an evaluation. NMST detected that the snack he was eating a couple of times a day was the culprit. After discussing with him, the offending snack was traced to the fig bar. Since he lived 40 miles from my office, since the fig bar was not available, I advised him to stay away from the fig bar for two days and return with it on the third day to get treated. His friend moved the box of fig bars from his bedside table to another room in order to keep it away from his electromagnetic field.

His friend was shocked at the discovery she made. There was only one bar left behind because he had eaten the rest in those weeks of his sickness. When asked, he said he did not have any appetite for other foods, so he lived on the fig bars during his sickness. By the time he returned to the office on the third day, he was feeling slightly better. The high fever was down. I treated him for the fig bar right away. The next day he reported that he had not had any more coughs, fever or wheezing after the treatment for fig bar. Whoever would suspect a fig bar (a healthy snack?) to cause pneumonia in a very healthy person? We all get fooled by these unsuspected allergens. Again, without the help of NMST, I wouldn't have tracked down the culprit.

People continue to suffer from various health problems and eventually, when their finances, spirits, motivation and hopes get exhausted, join the club of "Victims of Incurable Disorders." You can easily prevent something like that happening to you.

If you suffer from chronic asthma, when you visit a NAET specialist, he/she will begin treatments in the following order. The description of these allergens is given in my NAET Guidebook. It is available at our web-bookstore (www.naet.com) or at the Amazon.com bookstore.

If you see your NAET practitioner for any acute allergic attacks (asthma, bronchitis, pneumonia, sinusitis, etc.), if your practitioner is confident to treat an acute symptom, he/she may treat an allergen or a group of allergens out of the preferred order using the priority testing. If the practitioner is not experienced or not confident to treat an acute asthma problem, please call for emergency help by calling 911 if you are in the United States. When the acute symptom gets resolved, you can begin the treatment for the first allergen from the Basic-15 list, starting the following visit. NAET treatments can give quicker and more lasting relief if done properly and in the prescribed order. If not done properly, you may not get the desired results. After about 15 visits, if you don't see any improvement in your condition, you and your practitioner should get together and evaluate the situation.

NAET BASIC ALLERGENS GROUPS

The ingredients in the Basic allergen groups and what to avoid during the 25 hours following the treatment are given in the following pages. Information about these allergens in detail can be found in my book, "The NAET Guidebook." It is available at the NAET web bookstore, and at the amazon.com bookstore.

The Prescribed Order and what to eat or avoid for 25 hours following treatment:

1. BBF (brain, sympathetic and parasympathetic nervous system balance).

Nothing to avoid.

2. Egg mix (Egg white, egg yolk, tetracycline, chicken, feathers).

You may eat brown or white rice, pasta without eggs, vegetables, fruits, milk products, oils, beef, pork, fish, coffee, juice, soft drinks, water, and tea.

3. Calcium mix (breast milk, cow's milk, goat's milk, casein, albumin, and calcium).

You may eat cooked rice, (no raw fruits or vegetables) heated and cooled fruit juices, cooked vegetables (like potato, squash, green beans, yams, cauliflower, sweet potato), chicken, red meat, salt, oils, calcium-free water, coffee and tea without milk.

4. Vitamin C mix (fruits, vegetables, vinegar, citrus fruits, bioflavonoids, rutin, berries, vitamin C supplements, ascorbic acid, oxalic acid, citric acid).

You may eat cooked white or brown rice, pasta without sauce, boiled or poached eggs, baked or broiled chicken, fish, red meat, brown toast, deep fried food, French fries, salt, oils, and drink coffee or water.

5. B complex (B1, 2, 3, 4, 5, 6, 9, 12, 13, 15, 17, biotin, paba, inositol, choline).

You may only eat cooked white rice, white flour pasta, cookies and bread or pancakes made with white flour, cauliflower raw or cooked, well cooked or deep fried fish, salt, white sugar just for taste in a limited amount (no brown sugar or natural syrups), black coffee, French fries, and purified water when treating for any of the B vitamins. Rice should be washed well before cooking. It should be cooked in lots of water and drained well to remove the fortified vitamins. Since sugar is a helper of B vitamins, consuming too much sugar or eating sugary foods during the 25 hour period following B vitamins can cause treatment failure.

6. Sugar mix (cane sugar, corn sugar, maple sugar, grape sugar, rice sugar, brown sugar, beet sugar, fructose, molasses, honey, dextrose, glucose, and maltose).

You may eat white rice (white rice is pure starch, it is okay to eat since it takes time to convert into sugar; brown rice contains immediately available rice sugar in it), pasta, vegetables, vegetable oils, meats, eggs, chicken, water, coffee, tea without milk. Avoid fruits.

7. Iron mix (animal and vegetable sources: beef, pork, lamb, raisin, date, seeds, nuts, and broccoli).

You may eat white rice without iron fortification, sourdough bread without iron, cauliflower, white potato, chicken, light green vegetables (white cabbage, iceberg lettuce, white squash), yellow squash, and orange juice.

8. Vitamin A mix (animal and vegetable source, beta carotene, fish and shell fish).

You may eat cooked white rice, products made from white flour, pasta, potato, cauliflower, red apples, chicken, water, and coffee.

9. Minerals, water, drinking water, city water (magnesium, manganese, phosphorus, selenium, zinc, copper, cobalt, chromium, trace minerals, gold, and fluoride).

You may use only distilled water for washing, drinking, and showering. You may eat cooked rice, vegetables, fruits, meats, eggs, salt, oils, and drink milk, coffee, tea and distilled water. Avoid root vegetables (onions, potato, etc.).

10. Salt Mix (sodium and sodium chloride, table salt, sea salt, rock salt, iodized salt, water softener salts, and chemicals).

You may use distilled water for drinking and washing, cooked rice, cooked grains, fresh or cooked vegetables and fruits (except celery, and onions; avoid canned or preserved vegetables and vegetable products) meats, chicken, and sugar.

11. Grains (blue corn, yellow corn, cornstarch, corn silk, corn syrup; wheat, gluten, corn, oats, millet, barley, kamut, couscous, farina, and brown rice). In some cases you may be able to treat corn and grains together at one time. Please check with your practitioner for the possibility of treating together. In severe allergies, they should be treated separately. Avoid all products with gluten and grains.

You may eat steamed or cooked vegetables, white rice, fish, chicken, and meat. You may drink milk, water, tea and/or coffee. Avoid cream or sugar (corn may be a fortified ingredient in them).

12. Yeast mix, yogurt and whey (brewer's yeast, torula yeast, bakers yeast, candida, yogurt, whey).

You may eat rice, vegetables, fruits, meat, chicken, egg, turkey, beef, pork, beans, fish, and lamb. No fruits, no sugar products. Drink distilled water.

13. Stomach acid (Hydrochloric acid).

You may eat raw and steamed vegetables, cooked dried beans, eggs, oils, clarified butter, and milk.

14. Digestive enzymes (digestive juice from the intestinal tract contains various digestive enzymes: amylase, protease, lipase, maltase, peptidase, bromelain, cellulase, sucrase, papain, lactase, gluco-amylase, and alpha galactosidase).

You may eat acid producing foods: sugars, starches, grains, breads, and meats.

15. Hormones and Histamine (estrogen, progesterone, testosterone).

Histamine: Whenever there is an allergic reaction in the body, special cells (mast cells) release histamine. You can be allergic to your own histamine. When that happens, histamine is produced very frequently in the body. It doesn't stop until the mechanism is turned off. Another way to turn off histamine is to take antihistamine, either in a medication or a natural way by taking a large bolus dose of vitamin C (that is if you are not allergic to it). Ask your NAET practitioner about taking vitamin C to turn off histamine reaction. It is very easy to treat for your own histamine with NAET using a sample of histamine in the doctor's office. Then your body will stop abnormal histamine production with the exposure to every little harmless substance.

You may eat vegetables, fruits, grains, chicken, and fish.

HOME HELP FOR FOOD ALLERGIES

Collect a small portion of different foods from every meal and self-balance your points (Read Chapter 9) while holding the food mixture in a glass bottle (baby food jar will make an ideal sample-holder). Continue to do this for a month. Then collect samples from breakfast, lunch and dinner and treat the food mixture every night before going to bed. Continue this for six months to a year. When you stop having immediate reactions after eating, collect the food samples after each meal and keep in the refrigerator for 72 hours. If you had any delayed reaction, take the sample and self-treat or take it to your NAET practitioner for treatment. If you did not have any unpleasant reaction within 72 hours, most likely you are not allergic to the foods and can throw away the sample.

NAET CLASSIC ALLERGENS

The NAET Classic Allergens include the above 15 NAET Basic Allergens groups plus 40 other major allergen groups. There are a total of 55 major groups of allergens in NAET classic allergens. After the Basic allergens, the preferred order of treatments is given below. About 80 percent of one's allergic reactions towards substances will diminish if one clears 100 percent on all these allergens.

16. Cold
17. Heat
18. Humidity
19. Dampness

20. Dust/ dust mites

21. Smoking/nicotine

22. Pollens

22. Perfume mix/ flowers

23. Nightshade vegetables/vegetable mix

24. Animal epithelial/dander

25. Virus mix

26. Bacteria mix

27. Grasses/weeds

28. Formaldehyde

29. Chemical mix (Soap, Detergent, etc.)

30. Turkey/serotonin

31. Food coloring/food additives

32. Artificial sweeteners

33. Coffee, chocolate and caffeine

34. Spice mix 1 & 2

35. Vegetable fat & animal fat

36. Nut mix-1 & nut mix-2

37. Fish and shell fish

38. Amino acids 1 & 2

39. Whiten-all

40. Fluoride

41. Gum mix
42. Dried bean mix
43. Alcohol
44. Gelatin
45. Vitamin D
46. Vitamin E
47. Vitamin F (fatty acids)
48. Vitamin T (thymus)
49. R.N.A. & D.N.A.
50. Starch mix (Carbohydrates)
51. Parasites
52. Latex/plastics
53. Crude oil/synthetic materials, etc.
54. Immunizations/vaccinations/ drugs
55. Pesticides

TREATMENT BY PRIORITY

After completing the basic 15, your NAET practitioner will evaluate your progress and, if needed, plan your treatment by priority to help with your immediate health problem, for example: treat an allergen that will help with breathing, asthma, sinusitis, cough, bronchitis, pneumonia, etc. After the basic fifteen, the rest of the classic NAET allergen groups can be rearranged to help with the immediate problem. This is called "treatment by priority."

What is treatment by priority? Let us look at some examples:

- If your major complaint was "asthma," after completing the Basic 15, if your asthma is still not under control, your NAET practitioner will begin treating specific allergens related to triggering asthma. For example: Dust mix, grass-pollens, cold (ice cube), humidity, dampness, wind, air condition, exercise, emotions involved with asthma, etc.

- If you suffer from sinusitis, soon after you complete the basic 15, your practitioner will treat you for formaldehyde, house-cleaning chemicals, perfume, pillow, bed linen, fabric softeners, newspaper and ink, marker pens, liquid paper (white out), etc.

- If you or your child has asthma, after completion of Basic 15, your NAET practitioner will treat for dust mites, stuffed toys, plastic toys, coloring books, crayons, drinking water, school water, school books, breakfast items, soft drinks, candy bars, pollens, grass mix, weeds, perfume, secondary smoke, animal dander, epithelial, blanket, etc.

All these individual treatment will work better after clearing allergies for the NAET Basic 15 allergens–they are the essential nutrients that once cleared, will jump-start you on your road to health.

9

NAET Self-Balancing Tips

The purpose of this book is not to train a lay person in medical procedures. The real purpose of this book is to inform people about NMST and NAET allergy elimination treatment, so that asthmatic patients can learn about the availability of such a treatment and, if interested, can locate the appropriate medical practitioners with proper NAET training to help eliminate their allergy-related asthma. Please look for a qualified NAET specialist at the web site:

http// www.naet.com

Information regarding a few self-evaluation procedures, a few self-balancing tips to prevent asthma attacks, and a few self-balancing tips to handle unexpected emergencies, are described in the following pages. These points and techniques, when used properly according to the accompanying instructions, might help to monitor, reduce or control your presenting asthmatic symptoms in varying degrees.

Self-balancing applications are discussed in this Chapter, with illustrations. These balancing techniques are safe to use on people at any age and in any condition. These procedures can be safely used in balancing animals too. According to Oriental medical principle, when one maintains one's body in a balanced state, the body will not experience any illness or adverse reaction like asthma. Just by keeping the body in a balanced state, many people have reported that they were able to keep their asthma under control. Some have reported reduction in their allergy-related other health conditions as well.

But again I would like to make the reader aware that these are only energy balancing techniques and should not be confused with actual NAET treatments done with a trained NAET specialist. These balancing techniques will not replace the need for a trained practitioner. These techniques alone are not sufficient to permanently eliminate your asthma. These procedures, when used properly as described in the following pages, will help to improve your overall health, reduce asthma, allergies, and allergic conditions but will not eliminate your asthma.

SEEING A PULMONOLOGIST

First of all you need to find out the status of your asthma. You should consult a pulmonologist (an asthma specialist) to evaluate your condition. The asthma specialist will perform appropriate lung function studies to determine the severity of your asthma. He/she will also prescribe appropriate bronchodilator and other necessary medications to help reduce or control your asthma if you suffer from noticeable symptoms. If you presently suffer from asthmatic attacks, I strongly recommend you to see a pulmonologist and use the appropriate medication to keep your symptoms under control before beginning the NAET treatments. NAET works better when you keep your symptoms under control while receiving NAET treatments.

The next thing you need is to get a peak flow meter to monitor your asthma. Your pulmonologist will provide you and help you understand the proper usage of the peak flow meter and teach you how to record your reading.

WHAT IS A PEAK FLOW METER?

A peak flow meter is a simple, portable, inexpensive device that measures the rate at which a person can exhale. With asthma, sometimes you may feel your breathing is fine, but when you measure it with a peak flow meter, your lung function might be slightly decreased. A peak flow meter can help you determine if your breathing function is normal or not. This helps you understand the pattern of your asthma and helps you manage it better.

Asthma sufferers blow into them quickly and forcefully, and the resulting peak flow reading indicates how difficult it is to breathe out or how easily the air goes in and out of your lungs. In asthmatics, air gets trapped in the lungs (due to bronchial spasms) and the person is unable to breathe out the toxic air in order to breathe in fresh air. A peak flow meter can be used to determine the rate of air exchange and help you understand the following:

a. The severity of asthma;

b. Your response to treatment during an acute asthmatic episode;

c. The progress of treatment in chronic asthma cases;

d. The lung function on a daily basis without going through expensive testing procedures;

e. The level of lung function when exposed to known allergens. You can write down peak flow meter readings before and after exposure to allergens such as foods, drinks, dust mites, irritants such as cigarette smoke, exercise or disturbing emotional events.

Asthma is usually worse at night, although some patients sleep through the night unaware of lower peak flow levels. During sleep, normally there is a decrease in the amount of oxygen in the blood and this drop in oxygen may happen more often and last longer in people with asthma. You do not have to wake up at night to use the meter; simply compare your morning reading with your reading the night before to determine the degree of night asthma. A decrease of 15% or greater from the previous night's measurement may indicate nocturnal asthma. Peak flow readings fall before the symptoms of asthma are otherwise noticed. The earlier a warning sign is detected, the sooner the problem can be addressed.

HOW TO USE A PEAK FLOW METER

There are several steps for properly using a peak flow meter. You should blow hard on the meter to get the best reading possible, and repeat this attempt three times. Record the best of the three trials. All three measurements should be about the same to show that a good effort was made each time. This is especially important when parents are evaluating their child's asthma.

WHEN USING A PEAK FLOW METER:

- Make sure the device reads zero or is at base level.
- Take the reading in standing position if possible.
- Place the meter in your mouth and close your lips around the mouthpiece.
- Take a full deep breath.
- Blow out as hard and as fast as possible (one to two seconds).
- Do not cough or let your tongue block the mouthpiece.
- Write down the value obtained.
- Repeat the process two additional times, and record the highest of the three numbers in your chart.

It is also helpful to record readings before and after using inhaled bronchodilator if you are using one. Write all the readings each morning and night. Graphs for plotting peak flow readings often come with the devices and can be photocopied for further use. Take it to your doctor on each visit. Your doctor can gain a great deal of information by reviewing these readings. This also will help you to gain a better understanding of your lung function.

TESTING

In Chapter 6, you learned the NAET testing procedures to detect your asthma and allergies using NMST. You have learned to test and identify allergens in general that may be causing your asthma. Compare your NMST with the peak flow meter reading and you should record this finding also. If you want to keep your asthma under control, you are urged to practice these two testing techniques (peak flow reading and NMST) and make a habit of testing everything you suspect before exposing yourself to them. If you practice testing every item you come in contact with in your daily life, you will be surprised how soon you will become efficient in detecting each and every allergen that triggers your asthma. When you identify your allergens, you may be able to avoid them easily.

Commonly seen allergens around you are listed in Chapter 8. Please review the list of possible allergens around you.

Self-Testing Procedure # 1

HOLD, SIT AND TEST

Peak flow testing may not work for little children. The Hold, Sit and Test technique is an effective testing method for children. If learned correctly, this is easier than NMST to detect sensitivity to any allergen (also read Chapter 4). We teach this to our patients during patient-education class. Children are thrilled by this procedure. They can test secretly using this method for their food, cookies, drinks, clothes, etc., before parents get to test them with NMST.

Materials Needed:

1. A sample holder (thin glass jar, test tube, or a baby food jar with a lid can serve as a sample-holder).

2. Samples of the suspected allergens.

All perishable items, liquids, foods, should be placed inside the jar, then the lid should be closed tightly so that the smell will not bother the patient. If it is a piece of fabric, toy, etc., it can be held in the hand. Severe allergens like pesticides, perfume, chemicals, other toxic products should only be self-tested by adults, never by children.

PROCEDURE:

Place a small portion of the suspected allergen in the sample holder and hold it in your palm, touching the jar with the fingertips of the same hand for 15 to 30 minutes. If you are allergic to the item in the jar, you will begin to feel uneasy when holding the allergen, giving rise to various allergic symptoms or exaggerating the prior allergic symptoms. The intensity of symptoms experienced is directly related to the severity of the allergy. Please put away the jar as soon as you develop the uneasiness. Please do not wait until it becomes a full blown asthma.

When one holds an allergen, one or more of the symptoms from the following list may be experienced:

Abdominal discomforts
Anger
Asthma
Backaches
Begins to get hot or cold on various parts of the body
Blurry eyes
Brain fog
Butterfly sensation in the stomach
Chest pains
Cough
Craving
Crying spells

Deafness or ringing in the ear
Dry mouth, nose or throat
Fatigue
Flatulence
Frequency of urination
Headaches
Heaviness in the head
Heaviness in the chest
Heavy sensation in the body
Hives
Hyperactivity
Insomnia
Irregular heartbeats (fast or slow)
Irritability
Itching in the nose, eyes, cheeks and ears
Knee or other joint pains
Light-headedness
Migraine headaches
Mucus in the throat
Nausea
Nervousness
Nose bleeds
Pin prick sensation
Pins and needles on the palms or soles
Poor attention span
Poor bowel control
Poor vision
Rashes
Redness on the cheeks or ears
Restlessness
Runny nose or blocked nostrils
Shortness of breath
Sinus troubles
Sneezing attacks

Sudden appearance of canker sores
Sudden eruption of acne or pimples on the face or body
Suddenly becomes silent or suddenly becomes talkative
Unexplained pain anywhere in the body
Watery eyes
Weakness of any part of the limbs
Wheezing

Since the allergen is inside the sample-holder when such uncomfortable sensations are felt, the allergen can be put away immediately and the person can wash his/her hands to remove the energy of the allergen from the fingertips. This should stop the reaction immediately. In this way, you can test and determine allergens and the degree of your allergy towards them easily without putting yourself in danger.

NAET Testing Procedure #2

Testing and isolating a particular blockage can be done in many ways. One method, described below, is fairly easy to understand and, with some practice, can be mastered by anyone.

Subject and tester should wash their hands with soap and water before beginning the test, to remove any foreign energy from the fingertips.

Step 1: Balance the subject and find an indicator muscle. Refer to Chapter 6 to learn more about balancing and NMST.

Step 2: Patient lies down on his/her back with suspected allergen (e.g., an apple or item in sample-holder) in his/her resting palm. Lying down position will be easier and more reliable to perform this test. If a person cannot lie down, this can be done in seated position too. Use a surrogate when needed (to test an

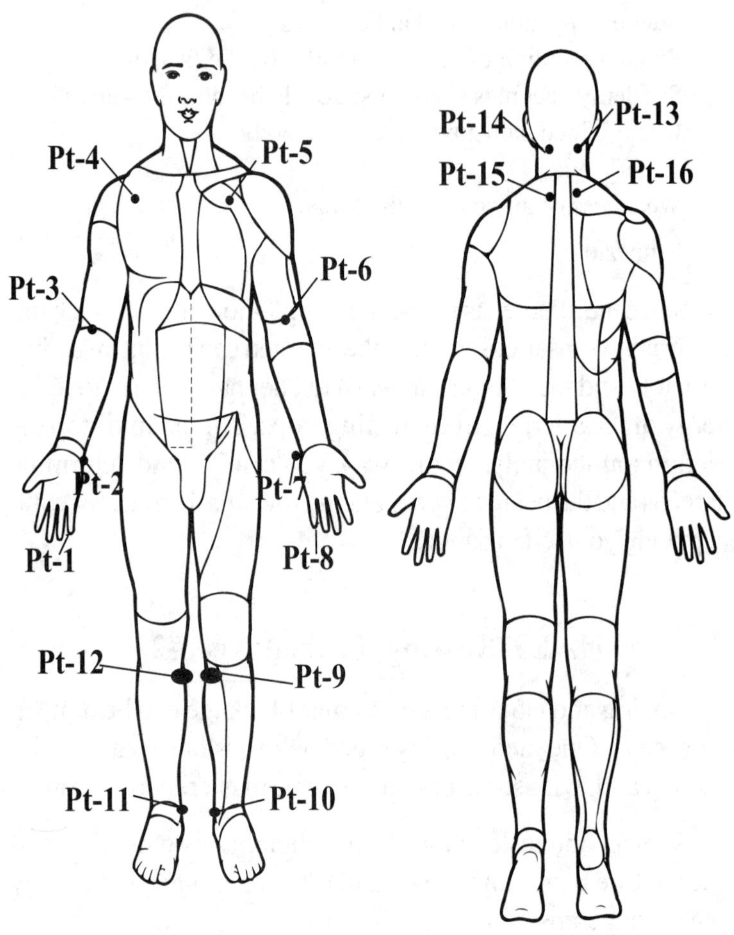

FIGURE 9-1
ASTHMA REDUCING POINTS

infant, a child, an invalid, a person in coma, a highly sensitive person, an animal, etc.)

Step 3: Tester touches the points in diagram 9-1 one at a time while testing the Pre-Determined Muscle (PDM) and compares the strength of the PDM in the absence and presence of the allergen. For example, touch point -1 in Figure 9-1 with the fingertips of one hand and with the other hand test the PDM (while the patient is still holding the allergen in one hand). If the test muscle goes weak, it indicates the meridian, or the energy pathways connected to that particular point, has an energy disturbance. Note: all these points do not belong to the lung meridian. Some are lung meridian points and capable of causing asthma; other points belong to other meridians that influence the lung function.

Points 1, 2, 7 & 8 belong to heart meridian. Heart meridian regulates the lung function.

Points 3, 4, 5, & 6 belong to the lung meridian.

Points 9 & 12 belong to spleen meridian. Spleen promotes the lung functions.

Points 10 & 11 belong to kidney meridian. Kidney balances the lung functions.

Points 13 & 14 belong to gall bladder meridian. This meridian controls the alveolar function, helping to empty and fill up the air sacs inside the lungs. These two points are very powerful and often can restore breathing in a respiratory arrest.

Points 15 & 16 are special acupuncture points, named "Free from Asthma." Together they regulate the breathing function of both lungs.

Point Name	Related Meridian	Related organ
Pt -1	Ht-9(Rt)	Heart
Pt - 2	Ht-7(Rt)	Emotional Heart
Pt - 3	Lu-5 (Rt)	Lung
Pt - 4	Lu-1 (Rt)	Lung
Pt - 5	Lu-1 (Lt)	Lung
Pt - 6	Lu 5 (Lt)	Lung
Pt - 7	Ht-7 (Lt)	Emotional Heart
Pt - 8	Ht-9(Lt)	Heart
Pt - 9	Sp 9 (Lt)	Spleen
Pt - 10	Kidney 3 (Lt)	Kidney
Pt - 11	Kidney 3 (Lt)	Kidney
Pt - 12	Sp-9 (Rt)	Spleen
Pt -13	GB-12 (Rt)	GB
Pt - 14	GB-12 (Lt)	GB
Pt - 15	Asthma Reduction point	(ARP-Lt)
Pt - 16	Asthma Reduction point	(ARP-Rt)

Table 9-1
Asthma Reducing Points (Front)

Test each point (shown in diagram 9-1) using this technique. Write down all the weak points. Using this technique, you can detect how severe the problem is. If only one point is weak, asthma is mild and will be reduced easily. If all twelve points are tested weak, the problem is extremely severe.

DESCRIPTION OF THE POINTS ON THE FRONT

Point 1: Ht-9 (Rt): On the thumb-side of the little finger, about 1/10 th of an inch posterior to the corner of the nail on the right.

Point 2: Ht-7(Rt): On the side of the little finger, at the end of the transverse crease of the wrist.

Point 3: Lu-5 (Rt):On the cubital crease, on the thumb-side.

point 4: Lu-1(Rt): Two finger-breadths below the acromial extremity of the clavicle, 6 finger-breadths lateral to the midline, (in the depression) on the right.

Point 5: Lu 1 (Lt): Two finger-breadths below the acromial extremity of the clavicle, 6 finger-breadths lateral to the midline, (in the depression) on the left.

Point 6: Lu-5 (Lt): On the cubital crease, on the thumb-side.

Point 7: Ht-7 (Lt): On the side of the little finger, at the end of the transverse crease of the wrist.

Point 8: Ht-9 (Lt): On the thumb-side of the little finger, about 1/10 th of an inch posterior to the corner of the nail.

Point 9: Sp-9 (Lt): On the lower border of the medial condyle of the tibia and M. gastrocnemius (below the knee joint on the front and medial side) on the left.

Point 10: Kid-3 (Lt): In the depression between the medial malleolus and tendocalcaneus, level with the tip of the medial malleolus on the left.

Point 11: Kid-3 (Rt): In the depression between the medial malleolus and tendocalcaneus, level with the tip of the medial malleolus on the right.

Point 12: Sp-9 (Rt): On the lower border of the medial condyle of the tibia and M. gastrocnemius (below the knee joint on the front and medial side) on the right.

DESCRIPTION OF THE POINTS AT THE BACK

Point 13: GB-12 (Rt): At the back of the head, in the depression posterior and inferior to the mastoid process on the right side.

Point 14: GB-12 (Lt):At the back of the head, in the depression posterior and inferior to the mastoid process on the left side.

Point 15: ARP (Lt): one finger breadth lateral to first thoracic vertebra, at the nape of the neck level with the shoulder on the left.

point 16: ARP (Rt):one finger breadth lateral to first thoracic vertebra, at the nape of the neck level with the shoulder on the right.

For Mild Asthma Cases Only

Anything other than mild cases should be evaluated appropriately by a well-trained NAET sp and a pulmonologist. Do not try to self-treat using these points if your case is serious. It is very dangerous to self-treat severe asthma symptoms without having the proper knowledge.

1. SELF-BALANCING PROCEDURE #1

Asthma Reducing Points

Any or all of these sixteen points shown in diagram 9-1 can be used to reduce or control asthma in mild cases. These points can be used to restore the energy flow in the respective meridians by removing energy interferences to improve lung function.

If you have mild asthma symptoms, use any one point from the right and another point from the left side of the body from diagram 9-1. First, gently massage (or tap) the point on the right for a minute. Then do the same on the left (for example: first massage clockwise or tap point 4 (Lu -Rt) for a minute, then point 5 (Lu-Lt) clockwise or tap for another minute). If you are still experiencing symptoms, continue three more times every ten minutes or until you feel better. Use all your medications if you have them with you. Using asthma medications is not contra indicated with NAET treatments provided you are not allergic to them. In fact, using them can help you pass the NAET treatments faster.

2. SELF-BALANCING PROCEDURE #2

Study the diagram 9-1. Balance the body twice a day using these points. Always finish the therapy at the first point where you started. If these points are used to reduce or control asthma, then do it every 20 minutes until you feel better, then continue once every two hours for rest of the day. The next day you can take rest. If you have another weak item, you may repeat the same procedure on the third day.

Step 1: The first step is to familiarize yourself with the test points. Then collect samples of each item you came in contact with or consumed 0-25 hours prior to your asthma attack. Test each allergen using NMST. Separate the allergens that made NMST positive (made the muscle weak on testing). Put away the ones that did not cause the muscle weakness. Then test the weak ones one at a time, touching each point in diagram 9-1 in the numerical order shown there. Write down all the weak NMST points. Find the related organs/meridians from table 9-1.

Step 2: Select the one that made your NMST weak while touching the points 4 or 5 (or both). Place that item in a glass container, hold the container in your one hand, and apply slight finger pressure with the pad of your index finger or have your partner or helper apply the finger pressure on your points. Start the acutherapy from the first point tested weak while testing. If the point-2 showed weak but not point-1, then start the balancing technique from point-2. Hold the point for 60 seconds. When you feel the pulsation under your finger pad (hold the point until you feel the pulsation), you can move on to the next point, following the numerical order.

Step 3: Hold 60 seconds at each point and go through all 15 points in the order given in figure 9-1 and finish the therapy at point-1 (beginning point). For example, after holding on the point-2, then go to point-3, then to point-4, 5, 6, 7, 8, 9, 10, 11, 12, 13, 14, 15, 16, 1 then again to point-2. The starting point is treated twice. So, hold 60 seconds at the starting point before stopping the treatment. Point-2 gets balanced twice. Always finish the therapy at the first point where you started.

If these points are used to reduce or control asthma, then do it every 20 minutes until you feel better, then continue once every two hours for rest of the day. The next day you can take rest.

If you have another weak item, you may repeat the same procedure on the third day.

SELF-BALANCING TECHNIQUE # 3

Backstroke Therapy for Infants and Children

Look at the Figure 9-2. Have the child lie on a flat surface (perhaps on a table). Support the child or hold the child with one hand over his/her back (either clothed or unclothed). Keep the allergen in a sample-holder near the child, touching an exposed area of the body. Gently stroke from neck down (Level-1) to level of the waistline (level-2) as shown in Figure 9-3. 13 strokes are applied at one cycle. Repeat the cycles every ten minutes until the child feels better or until help arrives.

After the acute phase is over, when the child's condition is stabilized, make an appointment with a NAET practitioner to get the NAET Basic 15 to 25 groups treated. Clearing the NAET Basic allergen groups will help prevent future similar attacks.

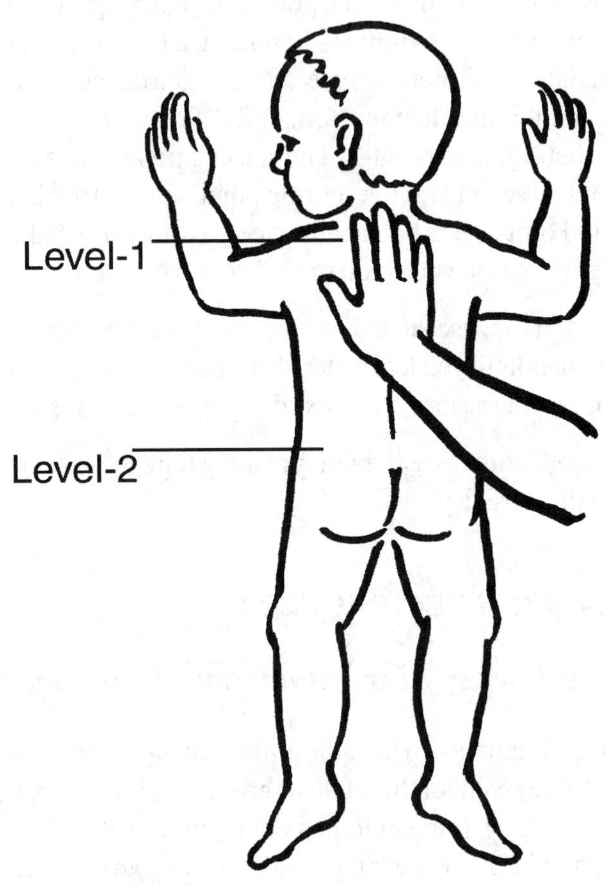

FIGURE 9-2
BACK-STROKE THERAPY

If you would like to learn more about acupuncture/ acupressure points or about meridians, please refer to the suggested textbooks in the bibliography. Chapter 10 in my book "Say Good-bye to Illness," may also help.

Acu therapy can help to keep your asthmatic symptoms under control.

It is a good idea to balance your body by applying Acu therapy or massaging the points clockwise, one minute on each point daily, twice a day. If you are very weak or sick, someone else can help to balance your points until you are strong enough to do so yourself.

You may also want to balance your points once or twice-a-day while you are going through NAET treatments with a practitioner. This will help you finish the treatments easier without having to repeat multiple times for the same allergen.

Who can use these self-balancing techniques?

You don't have to be sick to benefit from balancing the body. You can use balancing techniques with or without NAET treatments. Using these points you can never overbalance the body or overtreat the meridians. One can never be too healthy. If you are already healthy, you can maintain your health by doing acu therapy regularly. If you are sick, have allergies, or are unhealthy for whatever reasons, by treating these points regularly, you will feel better. Your immune system will improve if you maintain your body in a balanced state.

These NAET self-balancing techniques can also be used to balance the body not only in the morning or night, but any time you feel out of balance.

How do you know if you are out of balance?

If you are a healthy person, if your energy gets slightly out of balance you may not feel sick but may not feel quite right. You may feel tired, or sleepy in the afternoon, or may not have the right motivation to do your work, etc., but you cannot find a definite reason for such "out of sorts" feeling. Some minor energy disturbance in the meridians may be the cause. If you can immediately balance the body using these points, you will clear the energy blockage and feel normal in minutes.

Some patients can experience physical or emotional pain or an emotional release during these balancing sessions. If you remember any unpleasant memory from the past while massaging the points, continue to massage these points until you feel calm about the issue. Some patients can get tingling pains, sharp pains, pulsation, excessive perspiration, crying spells, etc., during the energy balancing session. In such instances, please go through another cycle of treatment. This will often correct the problem.

Learn to use the emergency help points. If you feel weak or sick, during the self-balancing session, please use the emergency help points. In spite of using those points, if you continue to feel sick, or if your asthma gets worse, please call for emergency help in USA by dialling 911.

Some commonly used acupuncture points, and their uses to help in emergency situations are given in the following pages. Knowing to use these points can save your life or someone you know. So, please take your time and learn them before you ever have an emergency situation.

ACUTE CARE

If a person is having an acute asthma (e.g. shortness of breath, cough, etc.), you can use acu therapy points to help bring the problem under control. Using the same method described above, massage these points and emergency points one minute on each point every ten minutes until the problem is resolved or until help arrives.

Children can get sick very easily. You may balance your child using self-help #2. Allergy may be the cause for the child's sickness. The usual culprits include: food, drinks, clothes, toys, etc.

Find the allergen causing the asthma, sinus congestion, shortness of breath, etc. by testing with NMST, using the information from Chapter 6. If you are able to trace the causative allergen, place the substance in a sample-holder, and have the child touch the sample-holder as you balance using # 2 method.

HANDLING ACUTE ASTHMATIC REACTIONS

If you get an acute asthmatic reaction to some food you ate in a restaurant or at home, or by coming in contact with an allergen, if you know the causative allergen, you may hold it in a sample-holder to balance your body using any of the three methods described above. You may repeat the balancing treatments ten minutes apart until you feel better. By treating this way, you may not clear the allergy permanently but you could control your asthmatic symptoms temporarily. When you stabilize your condition you should go to the appropriate medical practitioner for evaluation and further treatment.

As you have seen from the above description of energy balancing procedures, you can achieve good results by balancing acu-points on the front or back of the body. They both give similar results if done properly. When you balance your energy on your own, front acu-points are convenient to work with. But if you are helping someone else to balance his/her energy you may use the backstroke therapy technique, which can be applied to children as well as adults.

THE ORIENTAL MEDICINE CPR POINT

The CPR (cardiopulmonary rescuscitation) point of Oriental Medicine is the (GV-26) Governing Vessel-26.

Location: Below the nose, a little above the midpoint of the philtrum.

Indication: Fainting, sudden loss of consciousness, cardiac arrhythmia, heart attack, stroke, sudden loss of energy, hypoglycemia, heat stroke, sudden pain in the lower back, general lower backache, breathing problem due to allergic reactions, mental confusion, mental irritability, anger, uncontrollable rage, exercise-induced anaphylaxis, anaphylactic reactions to allergens, and sudden breathing problem due to any cause.

Procedure: Massage or stimulate the point for 30 seconds to a minute at the beginning of the problem.

- If you are treating yourself to wake up from sleeping while driving, or to recover from sudden loss of energy, etc., massage gently on this point. For example: While you are driving, if you feel sudden loss of energy or sensation of fainting, immediately massage this point. Your energy will begin to circulate faster and you will prevent a fainting episode.

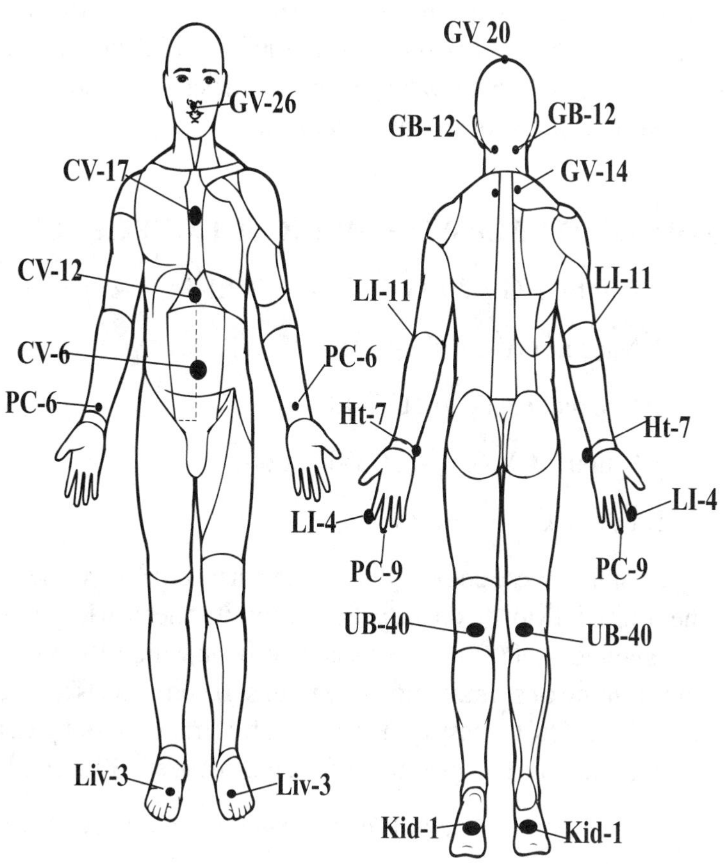

FIGURE 9-3

RESUSCITATION POINTS

- If you are reviving an unconscious victim who passed out in front of you, you may massage the point vigorously to inflict slight pain so that the person will wake up immediately. Vigorous massage is used only to wake up the fainted person or the person who became unresponsive in front of you.

POINTS TO HELP WITH MEDICAL EMERGENCIES

1. Fainting: GV-20, GV-26, GB-12, LI-1, PC-9, Kid-1
2. Nausea: CV-12, PC-6, Ht-7
3. Backache: GV-26, UB-40
4. Fatigue: CV-6, LI-1, CV-17, Liv-3
5. Fever: LI-11, GV-14

Stimulate these points by massaging them clockwise one at a time (from right to left on the patient's body) as needed to control acute symptoms. Patients will usually respond within 30 seconds to one minute of stimulating these points. If someone is slow to respond, it is OK to massage for three to five minutes. But please stop and evaluate the condition of the patient every 30 seconds.

Do not hesitate to call for emergency help (911), if you ever need it.

For more information on revival points, refer to Chapter 3, pages 570 to 573, in "Acupuncture: A Comprehensive Text," by Shanghai College of Traditional Medicine, Eastland Press, 1981, or refer to my book, "Living Pain Free with Acupressure," 1997, available at various bookstores and at our web site naet.com

GENERAL BALANCING TECHNIQUE

Look at the Figure 9-4. Massage these points gently for a minute each, clockwise, in circular motion with your fingertips starting from point-1, go through pt-2, pt-3, pt-4, pt-5,pt-6, and finish up the massage at point-1. A point stimulator may be used in place of finger massage. Massaging these points can improve the nerve energy circulation in the meridians. Treating these points will increase your overall energy. After each NAET treatment, these points should be massaged or needled to balance the body to help the NAET treatment last long.

HERBS WITH HEALING PROPERTIES:

1. Steam Inhalation to Clear Respiratory Passages

Preparation:

Use this steam bath, inhalation or fomentation on grown up children (over ten years old). For small children use the technique below.

In a large, heat proof bowl, pour steaming water. You can add nonallergic leaves, fresh flowers or dried, seeds, pollens, barks, tea bags, essential oils, essence, or tablets of the kind of herb you want to use. Add the flowers to the bowl when you pour the steaming water and keep it covered for 2 minutes before using the steam inhalation or bath. When you use oils or herbal essence

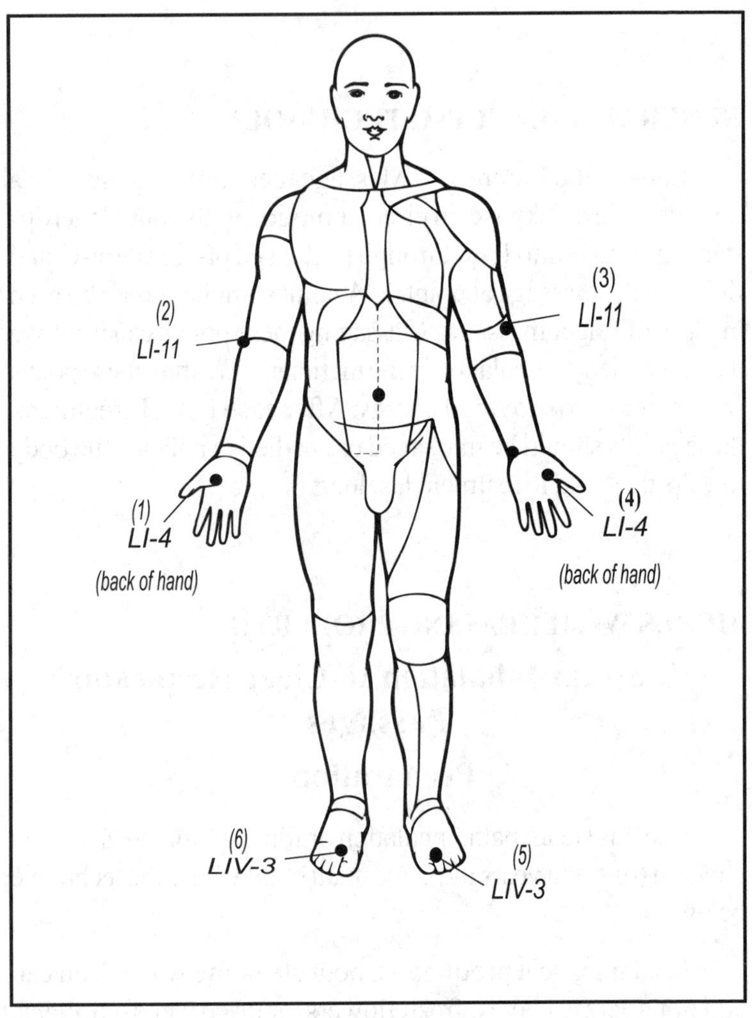

FIGURE 9-4
GENERAL BALANCING TECHNIQUE

let the water cool a little before adding the oil drops; otherwise the oils can evaporate quickly.

Create a tent by wrapping a bath towel around your head and drape it over the outer rim of the bowl. Sit with your face about 1 to 1 1/2 feet away from the bowl. Close your eyes and enjoy the relaxing steam. Take a few deep breaths. Try to inhale the steam through your nose and let it out through your mouth. Inhale the steam and allow the steam to penetrate your nasal passages, face, neck for about 10 minutes if you can tolerate; 3-5 minutes will be okay too. Avoid scalding or burning. Never do this on small children under ten. Never leave children unattended.

You can also use Vicks Vaporub or tablet, lemon barks, mint leaves, menthol, or lemon rind, instead of lemon leaves.

TECHNIQUE FOR LITTLE CHILDREN

For infants/ small children: Keep the pan with steaming water in the bathroom and seat the child or infant a few feet away from the pan. Close all the doors and windows. Open the lid completely and let the steam spread in throughout the room. Keep the child/infant away from the pan for 20 minutes. The vapor in the room will be sufficient to humidify the infant's lungs to loosen up the phlegm. You can also run the hot water for ten minutes in the bathroom with closed doors and windows. Then bring the child/infant in for five to ten minutes in the bathroom near the bowl with herbal water. This will help to fill up the room with steam faster.

HOW DOES IT WORK?

A steam bath is used in humidifying the respiratory passages and sinuses by stimulating the drainage of the mucus by opening up clogged up mucus-producing cells, sinuses and glands.

Indication: nasal congestion, shortness of breath due to common colds, influenza, reduce runny nose, cough and laryngitis followed by common colds. These herbs will work as therapeutic agents.

• Lemon leaves: Good to stop cough by opening up the nasal passages, throat, and larynx and eliminate phlegm.

• Cinnamon: Helps to improve energy in weak children who are too weak to cough up the phlegm. This is also helpful to prevent bad smell from the nasal passages due to clogged up old yellow, thick, mucus.

• Fresh ginger: To reduce pain.

• Menthol/Vicks and mint : Good to reduce sore throat.

• Hibiscus: Eliminate toxins.

• Lemon grass: Helps with pain in the face and sinuses.

• Fresh flowers of angel trumpet to reduce asthma (Datura Stramonia -

> You may add any of these in the steam inhalation to reduce the asthma or to clear respiratory passages.
>
> Basil
> Cedarwood
> Cypress
> Frankincense
> helichrysum
> hyssop
> Inula
> Lavander
> Lemon peel
> Myrrh
> Myrtle
> Valerian
> Violet
> Eucaluptus
> Oregano
> white flowers of angel's trumpet (Datura Stramonium)

white flowers are medicinal and the red flowers may cause hallucination).

After the steam inhalation, wrap the patient/child (especially the chest and neck area) with a warm blanket or scarf for 20 minutes. Give a warm drink to sip while sitting with the wrap.

Do it twice a day for a couple of days or more if you need it.

More Testimonials From Naet Patients

I suffered from sneezing and runny nose if I came near any dust. I had to wear a mask if I had to go out of the house. It was very embarrassing. My social life was limited. I took allergy shots since childhood. It helped me somewhat. I was referred to Dr. Devi by my chiropractor. After being treated for dust and dust mite with NAET, I do not react to dust anymore. I am able to travel all over the world now without wearing a mask. I visited India, Greece, Egypt and many European countries in the past couple of years without any trouble. NAET is a revolutionary technique indeed!

Dr. Toby Weiss
St. Croix, VI

Sinus Headaches and Allergic Rhinitis

I came to Doctor Devi a year ago with sinus headaches, shortness of breath, coughing, runny nose and wheezing. Within the first two months, my sinus headaches were reduced by almost 90 percent. The coughing and wheezing are virtually all gone. Now, we are working on eliminating allergy symptoms. I have been very pleased with her treatment and I have recommended her to many others.

Jim Ashley
Anaheim, CA

My Son's Asthma

My four-year old son was in one of his extreme asthmatic attacks, even using his face muscles to breathe—this after just having spent two hours on a hospital inhaler. Dr. Devi had me listen to his distressed lungs through a stethoscope and it was frightening! A few moments after one NAET treatment for water chemicals, we listened to his lungs again—and they were perfectly normal!

Vone Deporter
Woodland Hills, CA

Can Vitamin C Cause or Cure a Cold?

I was sold on Dr. Devi's treatment when I first got treated for Vitamin C. It seemed that I would get a cold once or twice a week and was still taking 2,000 or 3,000 units of vitamin C tablets a day. She found out I was allergic to vitamin C. I got treated, and now I feel better because I can absorb the vitamin C better.

Marla S.
Anaheim, CA

10

Allergies, Nutrition and Exercise

Vitamins and trace minerals are essential to life. They promote good health by regulating metabolism and assisting the biochemical processes that release energy from the foods and drinks we consume.

Vitamins and trace minerals are micronutrients, and the body needs them in small amounts. The lack of these essential elements, even though they are needed in minute amounts, can create various impairments and tissue damage. Water, carbohydrates, fats, proteins and bulk minerals like calcium, magnesium, sodium, potassium and phosphorus are considered to be macronutrients, taken into the body via regular food. They are needed in larger amounts. Both macro and micronutrients are not only necessary to produce energy for our daily bodily functions, but also for growth and development of the body and mind.

Using macronutrients (food and drinks) and micronutrients (vitamins and trace minerals), the body creates some essential chemicals — enzymes and hormones. These are the foundations of human bodily functions. Enzymes are the catalysts, or simple activators, in the chemical reactions that are continually taking place in the body. Without the appropriate vitamins and trace minerals, the production and function of the enzymes will be incomplete. Prolonged deficiency of these vitamins and minerals can produce immature or incomplete enzyme production, protein synthesis, cell mutation, immature RNA, DNA synthesis, etc., which can mimic various organic diseases in the body.

Deficiency of vitamins and other essential nutrients, can be due to poor intake and/or absorption. Nutritional imbalances can mainly be attributed to allergies. When your energy field conflicts with nutritional elements like vitamin C, calcium, B complex, etc., you cannot absorb the essential vitamins and minerals. The body cannot function properly lacking the enzymes and mediators, etc., which were to have formed in the presence of these vitamins and minerals. When the body does not produce complete enzymes, hormones and other immune mediators, your body will not proceed normally. The body malfunctions and continues to malfunction for a period of time; then temporary dysfunction can lead to major illness.

Vitamin and mineral deficiency syndromes can mimic many other organic diseases. When the body does not function properly, dysfunction will turn into disease. Desperate patients will start visiting professional health practitioners seeking relief for their problems. If nutritionists are consulted, they often place patients on large doses of various vitamins and minerals, along with certain health foods, some or all of which might not be absorbed due to allergy.

NUTRITIONAL DISORDERS

Many patients have nutritional deficiencies due to poor eating habits and will benefit from nutritional supplements and megavitamin therapy. Others may have nutritional deficiencies due to food allergies and will not show any improvements on vitamin therapy. In fact, most of these people will get worse. People who get well on vitamin therapy will consider it a miracle cure because once they fill up the deficiencies, their body functions will become normal. People who are allergic to certain vitamins and minerals cannot absorb them because their energy fields repel the energy fields of the vitamins and minerals. When regular food is eaten, a minute amount of vitamins and minerals are circulated through the body, creating minute fields and weak repulsion. But when a vitamin or mineral is taken in pill form, the concentration of the elements is greater than from food items, and so is the repulsion. This is possibly the reason why many allergic patients get very sick on vitamin/mineral therapy.

All patients should be tested for possible allergies before they are placed on vitamin therapy. If they are found to be allergic, they should be treated for the allergies before they are supplemented with vitamins and minerals, especially in mega-doses.

Apart from allergies, it is necessary to know a few things about taking vitamins and minerals. Of the major vitamins, vitamin C and B complex are water soluble, while vitamins A, D, E, and K are fat-soluble. It is believed that water-soluble vitamins must be taken into the body daily, as they cannot be stored and are excreted within one to four days.

When you are allergic to vitamin B complex, in many cases you cannot digest grains, resulting in B complex deficiencies. After you get treated for allergies via NAET, you can eat grains without any ill effect and will begin to assimilate B complex vitamins. In some cases, through NTT, I have found major B complex deficiencies. After NAET, then supplementing with large amounts of B complex for a few days to weeks as shown by NTT testing for vitamin dosage (5-10 times RDA amount per day for the specific number of days), the deficiency was eliminated. Over and over, in hundreds of patients, after weeks of supplementation, we have been able to remove their vitamin B complex deficiency symptoms completely. We have received similar results with vitamin C, but more research is needed on a larger number of patients to verify and prove these findings.

Fat-soluble vitamins are stored for longer periods of time in the body's fatty tissue and in the liver. When you are allergic to fat soluble vitamins, you begin to store them in unwanted places of the body. Some of this abnormal vitamin storage can be seen as lipomas, warts, skin tags, benign tumors inside the body or on the skin (boils or acne like small eruptions on the skin), etc.

Taking vitamins and minerals in their proper balance is important for the correct functioning of all vitamins. Excessive consumption of an isolated vitamin or mineral can produce unpleasant symptoms. High doses of one element can also cause depletion of other nutrients in the body, leading to other problems. Most of the vitamins work synergistically, complementing and/or strengthening each other's function.

Vitamins and minerals should be taken with meals unless specified otherwise. Oil-soluble vitamins should be taken before meals, and water-soluble vitamins should be taken during or after meals; however, when one is taking mega-doses of any of these, they should always be taken with or after meals. Vitamins and minerals, as nutritional supplements taken with meals, will supply the missing nutrients in our daily diets.

Synthetic vitamins are produced in a laboratory from isolated chemicals with quality similar to natural vitamins. Although there are no major chemical differences between a vitamin found in food and one created in a laboratory, natural supplements do not contain other unnatural ingredients. Supplements not labeled "natural" may include coal tars, artificial coloring, preservatives, sugars, and starches, as well as other additives.

These days, various nutrition books are available to help you understand vitamins and their assimilative processes. If anyone wants more information about nutrition, there are titles listed in the bibliography at the end of this book.

VITAMIN A

Clinical studies have proven vitamin A and beta-carotene to be very powerful immune-stimulants and protective agents. Vitamin A is essential for a variety of normal body functions. Its deficiency can cause disturbed lymphocyte production and function. A decreased lymphocyte production, or abnormal lymphocyte production, can cause decreased phagocyte activity, leading to lower immune function and autoimmune disorders.

Vitamin A is a wonder vitamin. It is necessary for proper vision, preventing night blindness, skin disorders, acne, to maintain healthy mucous membranes, etc., and it protects the body against colds, upper respiratory disorders, sinus troubles, dryness in the mucous membrane, influenza and other infections. It enhances immunity, helps heal ulcers, wounds, and maintains the epithelial cell tissue. It is necessary for the growth of bones and teeth. Vitamin A is an antioxidant that helps to eliminate endogenous toxins produced in the body from various adverse interactions taking place between the body and other foreign substances. Vitamin A protect the cells against cancer and other diseases.

Beta-carotene, from vegetable sources, converts into vitamin A in the liver, and is very good for cancer prevention.

Vitamin A helps in protein assimilation, slowing the aging process by building body resistance, fighting respiratory infections, promoting growth, maintaining clear, healthy skin, hair, nails, teeth and gums.

When you are allergic to vitamin A, or when vitamin A is not absorbed normally, vitamin A works adversely. The body perceives Vitamin A as an intruder and tries to throw it out when one tries to take more of it. If there is a problem with proper absorption and utilization of vitamin A, you can experience toxic symptoms such as poor or blurry vision, asthma, emphysema, shortness of breath, sinusitis, flu-like symptoms, repeated respiratory infections, lowered immunity, skin problems like rashes, boils, acne, skin tags, warts, unhealthy, wrinkled skin, premature aging, loss of hair and nails, unhealthy teeth and gums, headaches of various nature, infertility, irregular menses, pain in the joints, gastrointestinal disturbances like nausea, vomiting, diarrhea, indigestion, etc. If the allergy is treated, and if the diet is properly supplemented, the toxic symptoms can be completely eliminated.

Vitamin A works best with B complex, vitamin D, vitamin E, calcium, phosphorus and zinc. Zinc is needed to get vitamin A out of the liver, where it is usually stored. Large doses of vitamin A should be taken only under proper supervision because it can accumulate in the body and become toxic.

Food Sources: fish liver oil, milk and dairy products, butter, egg yolks, corn, green leafy or yellow vegetables, yellow fruits, liver, alfalfa, apricots, asparagus, beets, broccoli, carrots, Swiss chard, dandelion greens, garlic, kale, mustard, papayas, parsley, peaches, red peppers, sweet potatoes, spinach, spirulina, pumpkin, yellow squash, turnip greens and watercress.

Many teenagers who are allergic to vitamin A get acne, blemishes and other skin problems. Many people with allergy to vitamin A develop skin tags, warts, and pimples around the neck, arms, etc. This is also one of the causes of premenstrual syndrome. When people get treated and properly supplemented with vitamin A, the skin clears up and PMS problems become less severe.

VITAMIN D

Vitamin D is often called the sunshine vitamin. It is a fat-soluble vitamin, acquired through sunlight or food sources. Ultraviolet rays act on the oils of the skin to produce the vitamin, which is then absorbed into the body. Vitamin D is absorbed from foods, through the intestinal wall. Smog reduces the vitamin D-producing rays of the sun. Dark-skinned people and suntanned people do not absorb vitamin D from the sun. Vitamin D helps the utilization of calcium and phosphorus in the human body. It is important in the prevention and treatment of osteoporosis. It helps to improve the body's resistance against respiratory tract infections and helps to assimilate vitamin A. It also keeps skin and bones healthy.

When there is an allergy to vitamin D, the vitamin is not absorbed into the body through foods, or from the sun. People with an allergy to vitamin D can show deficiency syndromes such as rickets, severe tooth decay, softening of teeth and bones, osteomalacia, senile osteoporosis, sores on the skin, blisters on the skin while walking in the sun, severe sunburns when exposed to the sun, etc. Allergic persons can sometimes experience toxic symptoms if they take vitamin D without clearing its allergy. These symptoms include mental confusion, unusual thirst, sore eyes, itching skin, vomiting, diarrhea, urinary urgency, calcium deposits in the blood vessels and bones, restlessness in the sun, and inability to bear heat. Vitamin D works best with vitamin A, vitamin C, choline, calcium and phosphorus.

When an allergy to vitamin D is treated by NAET, the deficiency or toxic symptoms can be eliminated. With proper supplementation, normal health can be gradually restored.

Food Sources: fish-liver oils, dairy products fortified with vitamin D, alfalfa, butter, egg yolk, liver, sunshine, milk and milk products, meat, fish, eggs, cereal products, sweet potatoes, vegetable oils, beans, fruits and vegetables.

VITAMIN E

Vitamin E is an antioxidant that prevents cancer and cardiovascular disease. The body needs zinc in order to maintain proper levels of vitamin E in the blood. Vitamin E is a fat-soluble vitamin and is stored in the liver, fatty tissues, heart, muscles, testes, uterus, blood, adrenal glands and pituitary glands. Vitamin E is excreted in the feces if too much is taken. Even though it is fat-soluble, it is stored for only a short period of time in the body.

Among the numerous functions of vitamin E is its ability to suppress cellular aging due to oxidation. Vitamin E improves circulation, repairs tissue, treats fibrocystic breasts and premenstrual syndrome. It also promotes normal clotting and healing. It reduces scarring and blood pressure, helps prevent cataracts, leg cramps, age spots or liver spots. Because it is an antioxidant, and it protects the lungs against air pollution, supplying more oxygen to the body. It can help prevent or dissolve blood clots because it has an anticoagulant property. It promotes healing of minor wounds and skin irritation and can prevent scarring if applied topically. It has a big role in fertility. Vitamins E and A help the uterus prepare for pregnancy. Vitamin E aids in prevention of miscarriages, alleviates fatigue and helps to strengthen tired lower limbs after long walks or exercise. It also helps to reduce leg cramps by its vasodilation action and acts as a diuretic.

Deficiency syndrome includes destruction of red blood cells, muscle degeneration, some anemia, infertility, and heart and circulation problems. If you are allergic to vitamin E, you can show all the deficiency syndromes. After the proper elimination of vitamin E allergy, it can be supplemented for positive benefits.

Food Sources: vegetable oils, whole grains, dark green leafy vegetables, nuts, seeds, legumes, dry beans, brown rice, cornmeal, eggs, desiccated liver, milk, oat meal, organ meats, sweet potatoes, wheat germ, broccoli, brussels sprouts, spinach, enriched flour and whole wheat.

VITAMIN K

Vitamin K is needed for blood clotting and bone formation, and is necessary to convert glucose into glycogen for storage in the liver. Vitamin K is a fat-soluble vitamin, very essential to the formation of prothrombin, a blood-clotting material. It helps in the blood-clotting mechanism, prevents hemorrhages like nosebleeds and intestinal bleeding, and helps reduce excessive menstrual flow. An allergy to vitamin K can produce deficiency syndromes such as prolonged bleeding time, intestinal diseases like sprue, etc., and colitis.

Food Sources: alfalfa, broccoli, dark green leafy vegetables, soy beans, black strap molasses, brussels sprouts, cabbage, cauliflower, egg yolk, liver, oat meal, oats, rye, safflower oil and wheat. As mentioned earlier, allergy to vitamin K can cause blood-clotting disorders.

A four-year-old boy had been suffering from hemophilia since he was two years old. He bruised often in various joints, especially if he walked fast, ran or played with other children in school. Whenever he had an attack, he had to stay home with ice compresses on the affected joints for several days. He was found to be allergic to cabbage, a staple diet in his house. When he was treated for cabbage and vitamin K by NAET, his hemophilia-like symptoms disappeared. His family doctor declared him to be in remission. He is an active teenager now, without any trace of his previous symptoms.

VITAMIN B COMPLEX

Approximately 15 vitamins make up the B complex family. Each one of them has unique, very important functions. If the body does not absorb and utilize any or all of the B vitamins, various health problems can result. B complex vitamins are very essential for emotional, physical and physiological well-being of the human body. It is a nerve food, so it is necessary for the proper growth and maintenance of the nervous system and brain function. It also keeps the nerves well fed so that nerves are kept calm and the person maintains a good mental attitude. Certain B vitamins function as enzyme precursors and aid in digestion. The most important B vitamins and their function are:

B1- Affects the nervous system and mental attitude, aids in digestion of sugar and carbohydrates, helps to treat alcoholics and reduces stress by calming the nerves.

B2 - Aids in growth and reproduction. Promotes healthy skin, nails and hair, aids in digestion of carbohydrates, fats and proteins.

B6 - Aids in digestion and assimilation of proteins and fats, prevents various nervous and skin disorders, reduces morning sickness and nausea in general, promotes synthesis of nucleic acids, reduces neuralgia and neuritis, and works as a natural diuretic.

B12 - Prevents anemia, regenerates red blood cells, increases overall energy, maintains a healthy nervous system, aids in digestion of carbohydrates, fats and proteins, improves concentration, memory and emotional balance.

FOLIC ACID

Essential to the formation of red blood cells and prevents anemia; aids in protein metabolism and production of nucleic acids; helps in cell division, essential for utilization of sugar and amino acids; improves lactation, delays hair graying when used with PABA and pantothenic acid.

BIOTIN

Water soluble, required in trace amount. Usually measures in micrograms (mcg.). Vitamin C synthesis requires biotin. Essential for normal metabolism of fat and protein. It promotes healthy skin and hair, ease muscle pain, helps remove dermatitis, eczema and shortness of breath. It can be synthesized by intestinal bacteria. Raw eggs prevents absorption in the body.

Food sources: Nuts, fruits, brewer's yeast, beef liver, egg yolk, milk, kidney, unpolished rice.

INOSITOL

Promotes healthy hair and prevents hair loss, aids in redistribution of body fat, lowers cholesterol, produces a calming effect. Inositol, choline, pantothenic acid and B12 taken together help improve concentration and memory.

Allergic symptoms can appear in many forms if one is allergic to B vitamins. The doctor has to take special care to isolate the allergic vitamin and treat to alleviate the problem. B vitamins are seen in almost all foods we eat. Some B vitamins are destroyed by cooking and heating, some are not destroyed by processing or preparation. People who are allergic to B vitamins can get mild to severe reactions just by eating the foods alone. If they are supplemented with vitamin B complex, if they are not aware of their B complex allergy., such people can get exaggerated reactions. One has to be very cautious while taking B complex.

Food sources of B vitamins include whole grains, seeds, legumes, milk products, pork, liver, beef, green leafy vegetables, potatoes, nuts, eggs, fish, root vegetables, green vegetables, fruits, brewer's yeast, bran and wheat germ.

Dr. Carlton Frederick, in his book, Psychonutrition, tried to point out that nutritional deficiencies are the causes of most of the mental sicknesses in psychiatric facilities. He tried to prove his theory by giving large doses of vitamin B complex, especially B12, to some of the psychiatric patients. Fifty percent of the patients were cured of their mental sickness and went back to live normal lives. But the other 50 percent made no progress or got worse. So his theory was thrown out, his book was banned from circulation and he was ridiculed. When I discovered NAET, I tried to contact Dr. Frederick to inform him the possible reason behind the unresponsive 50% to his B12 vitamin treatment was an allergy. Unfortunately he had passed away one year before my search to find him. He never had the destiny to find out that he was right about the connection between nutritional deficiencies and mental illnesses.

VITAMIN C

Vitamin C, or ascorbic acid, is a water soluble vitamin that plays a very important role in the metabolism of carbohydrates, proteins and lipids. Vitamin C is fairly stable in acid solution. It is very sensitive to oxygen. Its potency can be lost through exposure to light, heat and air.

Vitamin C is readily absorbed through the mucosa of the mouth, stomach and mostly through the upper part of the small intestine. From there, it passes through the portal vein to the liver and is distributed to tissues throughout the body. The transport mechanism may differ from person to person. The level of ascorbic acid in the blood reaches a maximum in two or three hours after ingestion, then decreases as it is eliminated in the urine and through perspiration. Most of the vitamin C is out of the body within three or four hours.

To maintain an adequate serum level, this vitamin should be taken in small amounts throughout the day. A human body stores a total of about 1,500 milligrams with moderate reserves in the liver and spleen, and high concentration in the adrenal glands.

Vitamin C is essential in the formation of adrenaline. During stress, the adrenals use vitamin C rapidly. For this reason, more vitamin C is needed under stressful conditions. Vitamin C helps in preventing scurvy. Vitamin C promotes fine bone and tooth formation while protecting the dentine and pulp. It reduces the effects on the body of some allergy-producing substances. In large doses, it can function as antihistamine and reduce allergic reactions. Allergic patients benefit from taking adequate amounts of vitamin

C every day to reduce their various reactions, but must make sure they are not allergic to the vitamin C products they are taking.

Vitamin C is used in the prevention of the common cold. It is an important nutrient in treating wounds because it speeds up the healing process. It is very important in the formation of collagen, a major component of all connective tissues: skin, bones, teeth, muscles, tendons, etc. Vitamin C is necessary to transport certain amino acids, such as proline and lysine, into hydroxy proline and hydroxy lysine. These hydroxy forms give stability to the collagen molecules.

Vitamin C prevents breakdown of connective tissue. It helps amino acids in the synthesis of neurotransmitters. It also helps with the absorption of iron and helps in various enzymatic functions in the body. It helps improve the healing of wear and tear of the tissues. It nourishes the tissues of the blood vessels and helps improve their elasticity. Healthy blood vessels improve blood circulation. Efficient blood circulation helps to reduce serum cholesterol. Good circulation also gives good elimination; thus vitamin C helps with constipation.

Elimination of the toxins from the body brings about a good complexion. Vitamin C also helps to maintain the water balance in the body by redistributing or removing excess amounts of water; this is an essential vitamin in weight control, a good antioxidant, seen in almost all foods. Overcooking destroys it.

An allergy to Vitamin C can cause severe asthma which does not respond to any therapies.

MINERALS

A few minerals are extremely essential for our daily functions. While some metals and trace minerals are mentioned here, please refer to the appropriate references in the bibliography for more information on other minerals.

CALCIUM

Calcium is one of the essential minerals in the body. Calcium works with phosphorus, magnesium, iron, vitamins A, C and D and helps to maintain strong bones and healthy teeth. It regulates heart functions and helps to relax nerves and muscles. It induces relaxation and sleep.

Deficiencies in calcium can result in rickets, osteomalacia, osteoporosis, hyperactivity, restlessness, inability to relax, generalized aches and pains, joint pains, formation of bone spurs, backaches, PMS, cramps in the legs, and heavy menstrual flow.

Food sources for calcium are milk products, soybean, sardine, oyster, salmon, nuts, dried beans and green leafy vegetables. If you are allergic to calcium, you can get deficiency syndromes in exaggerated forms whenever you eat foods containing calcium. When the allergy is eliminated by NAET, you can be supplemented appropriately to get maximum health benefits.

Many asthmatics with upper respiratory problems respond well to calcium supplementation. Many people with abdominal pains, dysentery, insomnia, skin problems, nervousness, dyslexia, canker sores, postnasal drip, hyperactivity, obesity, and arthritis respond well to allergy treatments for calcium and, later, supplementation. Many women who have heavy menstrual flow respond well to allergy treatment for calcium and later supplementation. When people are on cortisone treatment, they need to take more calcium.

IRON

Iron is one of the essential minerals, necessary for the production of hemoglobin (red blood corpuscles), myoglobin (red pigment in muscles), and certain enzymes. In one month, menstruating women deplete more iron than men. Iron requires copper, cobalt, manganese, and vitamin C for proper assimilation. It is also necessary for proper metabolizing of B vitamins. Iron aids in growth, promotes resistance to disease, prevents fatigue, prevents and cures iron deficiency anemia.

Iron deficiency results in anemia. People with allergy to iron do not absorb iron from food. They suffer from iron deficiency anemia, even though they take iron supplements. A person with iron allergy can have various problems due to iron supplementation or/from eating iron-containing foods.

Food sources: apricots, peaches, bananas, black strap molasses, prunes, raisins, brewer's yeast, whole grain cereals, spinach, beets, alfalfa, sunflower seeds, walnuts, sesame seeds, dried beans, lentils, liver, egg yolk, red meats, pork, kidney, heart, clams, oysters, oat meal and asparagus.

CHROMIUM

Chromium is an essential element to metabolize sugar, and to treat diabetes, hypoglycemia, and alcoholism. A deficiency results in arteriosclerosis, hypoglycemia, shortness of breath, and diabetes.

Food sources: whole grain cereals, wheat germ, corn oil, brewers' yeast, mushroom, liver, raw sugar, red meat, shellfish, chicken and clams.

COBALT

Cobalt is essential for red blood cells since it is part of vitamin B12. Deficiency results in B12 deficiency anemia.

Food sources: all green leafy vegetables, meat, liver, kidney, figs, buckwheat, oysters, clams and milk.

COPPER

Copper is required to convert the body's iron into hemoglobin. Combined with the amino acid thyroxin, it helps to produce the pigment factor for hair and skin. It is essential for utilization of vitamin C. Deficiency results in anemia and edema. Toxicity symptoms are insomnia, hair loss, irregular menses and depression.

Food sources: almonds, beans, peas, green leafy vegetables, whole grain products, prunes, raisins, liver, dried beans, whole wheat, beef, most seafood, and copper piping in water supply.

FLUORINE / FLUORIDE

Sodium fluoride is added to drinking water. Calcium fluoride is seen in natural food sources. Fluorine decreases chances of dental carries (too much can discolor teeth). It also strengthens the bones. Deficiency leads to tooth decay. Toxicity or allergy symptoms include dizziness, nausea, poor appetite, skin rashes, itching, yeast infections, mental confusion, muscle spasms, mental fogginess and arthritis. Treatment for fluoride will eliminate possible allergies. Food sources include fluoridated drinking water, seafood, gelatin, sunflower seeds, milk products, carrots, garlic, green leafy vegetable and almonds.

IODINE

Two-thirds of the body's iodine is in the thyroid gland. Since the thyroid gland controls metabolism, and iodine influences the thyroid, an under-supply of this mineral can result in weight gain, general fatigue and slow mental reaction. Iodine helps to keep the body at a correct weight, promotes growth, gives more energy, improves mental alertness, and promotes the growth of hair, nails and teeth.

A deficiency in iodine can cause overweight, hypothyroidism, goiters, lack of energy and shortness of breath.

Food sources: kelp, seafood, iodized salt, vegetables grown in iodine-rich soil and onion.

MAGNESIUM

Magnesium is necessary for the metabolism of calcium, vitamin C, phosphorus, sodium, potassium and vitamin A. It is essential for the normal functioning of nerves and muscles. It also helps convert blood sugar into energy. It works as a natural tranquilizer, laxative and diuretic. Diuretics deplete magnesium. Alcoholics and asthmatics are deficient in magnesium.

Food sources: nuts, soybeans, raw and cooked green leafy vegetables, almonds, whole grains, sunflower seeds, brown rice and sesame seeds.

MANGANESE

Manganese helps to activate digestive enzymes. It is important in the formation of thyroxin, the principal hormone of the thyroid gland. It is necessary for the proper digestion and utilization of food. Manganese is important in reproduction, and in the normal functioning of the central nervous system. It helps to eliminate fatigue, improves memory, reduces nervous irritability and relaxes the mind. A deficiency may result in recurrent attacks of dizziness and poor memory.

Food sources: green leafy vegetables, spinach, beets, brussels sprouts, blueberries, oranges, grapefruits, apricots, the outer coating of nuts and grains (bran), peas, kelp, egg yolks, wheat germ and nuts.

MOLYBDENUM

Molybdenum helps in carbohydrate and fat metabolism. It is a vital part of the enzyme responsible for iron utilization.

Food sources are whole grains, brown rice, brewer's yeast, legumes, buckwheat, millet and dark green leafy vegetables.

PHOSPHORUS

Phosphorus is involved in virtually all physiological chemical reactions in the body. It is necessary for normal bone and teeth formation. It is important for heart regularity, and is essential for normal kidney function. It provides energy and vigor by helping in the fat and carbohydrate metabolism. It promotes growth and repairs in the body. It is essential for healthy gums and teeth. Vitamin D and calcium are essential for its proper functioning.

Food sources: whole grains, seeds, nuts, legumes, milk products, egg, fish, corn, dried fruits, poultry and meat.

POTASSIUM

Potassium works with sodium to regulate the body's water balance and to regulate the heart rhythm. It helps in clear thinking by sending oxygen to the brain. A deficiency in potassium results in edema, hypoglycemia, nervous irritability, and muscle weakness.

Food sources: all vegetables, especially green leafy vegetables, oranges, whole grains, sunflower seeds, nuts, bananas, potatoes, potato peelings, citrus fruits, melons, tomatoes, watercress and mint.

SELENIUM

Selenium, an antioxidant, helps asthmatics to eliminate endogenous toxins. It works with vitamin E, slowing down the aging process. It prevents hardening of tissues and helps to retain youthful appearance. Selenium is also known to alleviate hot flashes and menopausal distress. It prevents dandruff. Some researchers have found selenium to neutralize certain carcinogens and provide protection from some cancers.

Food sources: brewer's yeast, wheat germ, sea water, kelp, garlic, mushrooms, seafood, milk, eggs, whole grains, beef, fish, beans, most vegetables, bran, tuna fish, onions, tomatoes and broccoli.

SODIUM

It is essential for normal growth and normal body functioning. Poor absorption and utilization of sodium chloride can cause asthma and water retention in the lungs. It works with potassium to maintain the sodium-potassium pump in the body. Potassium is found inside the cells and sodium is found outside. It is essential to maintain processed foods including most fast foods. Many food additives include sodium and food additives like sodium nitrates may cause high blood pressure in sensitive people.

Food sources: salt, shellfish, carrots, celery, beets, artichokes, beef, brain, kidney and bacon.

SULFUR

Sulfur is essential for healthy hair, skin and nails. It helps maintain the oxygen balance necessary for proper brain function. It works with B complex vitamins for basic body metabolism. It is a part of tissue building amino acid. It tones up the skin and makes the hair lustrous and helps fight bacterial infection.

Food sources: radishes, turnips, onions, celery, string beans, watercress, soybean, fish, meat, lean beef, dried beans, eggs, cabbage, grapes, raisins, dried foods, wines, alcoholic beverages, saccharin, Sweet and Low, sulfites and sulfates.

VANADIUM

Vanadium prevents heart attacks. It inhibits the formation of cholesterol in blood vessels.

Food sources: all fish, seaweed, dark green vegetables, vegetables grown near the ocean.

ZINC

Zinc is essential to form certain enzymes and hormones. It is necessary for protein synthesis. It is important for blood stability and in maintaining the body's acid-alkaline balance. It is important in the development of reproductive organs and helps to normalize the prostate glands in males. It helps in treatment of mental disorders and speeds up healing of wounds and cuts on the body. Zinc helps with the growth of fingernails and eliminates cholesterol deposits in the blood vessels.

Food sources: Wheat bran, wheat germ, pumpkin seeds, sunflower seeds, brewers' yeast, milk, eggs, onions, green leafy vegetables, oysters, herring, peas, brown rice, fish, mushrooms, lamb, beef, pork, nonfat dry milk and mustard.

TRACE MINERALS

Even though trace minerals are needed in our bodies, they are needed in minute amounts only. The researchers do not know the definite functions of the trace minerals, but deficiencies can definitely contribute toward health problems. Their food sources include alfalfa, kelp, seafood and seawater.

AMINO ACIDS

All proteins are made up of amino acids. They are the building blocks of protein. There are 22 amino acids. Some can be made in the body and are called nonessential amino acids. Eight are not produced in the body and are known as essential amino acids. These essential amino acids that have to be absorbed from food are lysine, methionine, leucine, threonine, valine, tryptophan, isoleucine and phenylalanine. Children also need histidine and arginine.

When people are allergic to amino acids, they suffer from various protein deficiency and protein metabolism disorders. Some of the genetic disorders or errors of protein metabolism can be reversed when treated with NAET for each individual amino acid (Cystic fibrosis, certain chromosomal disorders, etc.).

Food sources: protein foods (meat, fish, poultry and dairy products), nuts, beans, dried beans, etc. Most vegetables, grains and fruits are incomplete proteins. But when they are taken in combination, such as legumes with grains, they can provide complete proteins.

LECITHIN

Lecithin is needed by every living cell in the human body. Cell membranes which are largely composed of lecithin, select and regulate which nutrients may leave or enter the cell. Cell membranes would harden without lecithin. Its structure protects the cells from damage by oxidation. The protective sheaths surrounding the brain are composed of lecithin, and the muscles and nerve cells also contain this essential fatty substance. Lecithin is composed of choline, inositol and linoleic acids. It acts as an emulsifying agent.

It helps prevent arteriosclerosis, protects against cardiovascular disease, increases brain function, and promotes energy. It promotes better digestion of fats and helps disperse cholesterol in water and removes it from the body. The vital organs and arteries are protected from fatty buildup with the inclusion of lecithin in the diet. Most lecithin is derived from soybean, eggs, brewer's yeast, grains, legumes, fish and wheat germ.

If an allergy to lecithin is eliminated and it is assimilated in the body from your daily food, the body will be able to normalize the blood serum cholesterol, which can help overall circulation.

From this information, the reader may gain an understanding of the importance of good nutrition (non-allergic nutrients) to maintain a proper balance of the body's functions. The body needs all the essential vitamins and minerals in proper proportion for its normal function. Deficiency of vitamins, minerals, trace minerals, or amino acids can manifest as functional disorders or other problems. If deficiency can be found in time and treated or supplemented in appropriate amounts, many unnecessary discomforts can be avoided.

The important supplements to strengthen the respiratory system should include: Calcium, magnesium, boron, biotin, L-glutamine, L-proline, L-Lysine, Taurine, zinc, manganese, vitamin A, vitamin E, vitamin C, vitamin B6, vitamin B12, selenium, citrus bioflavonoids, fatty acids, hydrochloric acid, amylase, lipase, cellulase, bromelain, lactase, chromium, B complex and trace minerals.

SUPPLEMENTATION

This can also be used to test for adequate dosages of medications, adequate amount of daily food, number of servings of food groups, slices of bread to be eaten daily, ounces of meat or protein to be eaten, etc. Your NAET doctor can help you to find all these. He/she can teach you how to do it yourself so that you will be able to test yourself and adjust the daily dosages (amounts) on your own.

GOOD NUTRITION

Now you have learned to test your allergies, and to eliminate your allergies to foods, nutrients, environments, and other products you use in your life. After going through the NAET program, you will finally reach your goal. Now you can eat anything you want to, use anything you like to without causing asthma or other respiratory disorders. You have found your freedom to breathe, to live again as a normal person. Now it is your job to maintain your health by nourishing your body adequately, helping the body eliminate the endogenous toxins as they build up in your body. Eating sensible, healthy and nutritious meals are important to maintain the health you received with great effort, so is adequate exercises.

WATER INTAKE

Most health advisories stress drinking adequate amounts of water. How much is adequate? I have not seen correct information in many places. When I studied nutrition in school, my teacher gave this formula for drinking water. It works well for most people: Take your weight in pounds, divide it by two, and drink that many ounces of nonallergic water daily. If you weigh 100 pounds, then half of that is 50. So, 50 ounces of water a day is your required daily amount of water.

There is no one specific kind of water safe to drink or use. If you drink water to which you are allergic, it can do more harm than good. Bottled water is not always safe. I have found that bottled water causes a great many problems in many people due to allergies. Try to test your water before you drink it or use it for washing, etc. If you found an allergy to the water, please treat it before you use, or find another kind. There are many brands available. If you learn to test properly, you will find some nonallergic ones in the market place.

You may also use water filters. Make sure to use reliable filters. A few years ago, when I was reacting to every kind of bottled water, I decided to get a whole house water filter. I tried a few brands but I was not satisfied because I was still reacting to the water filtered through these special (some very expensive) filters. After many trials and discouragements, finally, about ten years ago, I found the Culligan water filter. I have not reacted to water ever since. So I highly recommend the Culligan water filter system. But everyone's reactions are different. What works for one person might not work for someone else.

TIME TO DRINK

It is good to spread it through the day. But if it is inconvenient, you may drink at any time. As long as you drink the required ounces a day, your body can eliminate the impurities conveniently. When you drink large amounts of water you may need to urinate frequently. If your schedule does not permit that, you can drink the water in the evening when you have more time to relax. Some people might say that their sleep might get disturbed if they drink too late. If you are afraid of that try to drink the major part of your water before 6:00 p.m. When you clear all known allergies, sleep disturbance may not be a problem. If you wake up in the middle of your sleep to urinate, you will be able to get back to sleep soon after.

Some people may not like drinking water at all. Some have said they are not thirsty. These people probably have more allergies to clear. Their spleen meridian is probably underactive. If they can eat four ounces of dried red cherries daily that will improve the health of the spleen meridian and they will be able to drink the required amount of water, utilize it and eliminate impurities as desired.

Some people may not like the taste of plain water. You may add a drop of mint extract, cinnamon extract, lemon grass extract, ginger extract, cumin seed extract, or a few drops of fresh lemon juice to the water to make it taste better. Water can also be drunk as hot teas or iced teas. Coffee or fruit juice is not a substitute for drinking water.

THE RIGHT FOOD

All nonallergic food is right for you. Regular store-bought food and health food store-bought food have similar benefits as long as you are not allergic to them. But if you are allergic to the food, no matter where you bought it, you are going to get sick. Pesticide content is higher in foods from a regular store. If you eliminate allergy to pesticides, your body will be able to eliminate the incoming pesticides naturally. But your body has to work more to eliminate the toxins from pesticides. When you consume less pesticides, your body has to work less to eliminate the toxins. When produce is grown organically, the general nutrition content is better. But wherever you buy, you must test your reactivity to foods before you use them.

While going through early NAET treatments, you are required to eat nutrition-depleted foods like: washed out white rice, white pasta, inside of the potato, French fries, cauliflower, lettuce, etc. The purpose of eating a diet that has less nutrition during treatments is to prevent treatment failure due to the exposure to nutrients. But soon after completing the required avoidance time on each early treatment, you should include a healthy, balanced diet in your everyday menu. Your daily diet should be selected wisely from the list given below to provide adequate nutrition. Your food can strengthen or weaken your immune system. You can select specific foods to strengthen your meridians, body, and the immune system. It will be beneficial to choose your foods according to your own body's requirement.

THE RIGHT AMOUNT

After clearing the allergies, some of my patients began eating without stopping. Their excuse was that they were never free to eat all they wanted before and now since they have the freedom, they like to eat to their satisfaction. Some people may eat a lot soon after they finish the treatment, then after a few weeks slow down. If they have problem slowing down, it is an indication that they are deficient in essential nutrients. Once the nutritional needs are met, the craving diminishes, and a small amount will satisfy the appetite.

You can check the amount of food your body needs using NAET Nutrient Supplementation Protocol.

FOODS FOR YOUR LUNGS

According to Eastern medical principles, one should blend all five flavors and prepare the meal each time. This is to nourish the entire body. The five flavors are effective not only upon the five viscera but upon all parts of the body that are connected with the viscera. *"If people pay attention to the five flavors and blend them well, their bones will remain straight, their muscles will remain tender and young, breath and blood will circulate freely, the pores will be fine in texture, and consequently breath and bones will be filled with the essence of life."* Nei Ching (Chinese Internal medicine text book). That is the description of normal health.(See Table 10-3).

If one part or organ is diseased, you need to nourish that organ to full health first, then you can maintain the health of the whole body. For example: when you have asthma, or other respiratory problems, your lung meridian is the weak one. Lung organ is only a small projection of the lung meridian. So find the foods that will strengthen your lungs. The commonly seen foods that nourish the lung meridians and organs are given in Tables 10-1 and 10-2. While you are getting NAET treatments and during the recovery period, if you provide your body with adequate nutrition, your recovery will be faster. Try to consume the major por-

List of foods to strengthen Lungs and Resp. System

This group gives flavoring to foods	Energy dispersing from lungs
	Pungent
Meats	Turtle, duck
Grains	Rice-brown, wild
Veg. proteins	Lentils, horse gram
Fruits	Orange, lemon, tangarine, pineapple,
Leafy vegetable	Onions , mint, parsley, cilandro
Root vegetable	Celery root, turnip, daikon
Hardy vegetable	zucchini, squah, asparagus
Veg. fats	Musturd oil, linseed oil, oregano oil, olive oil
Ani. fats	Fish oil, cheese, cl.butter
Nuts	Pine nut, cashew nut
Spices	Cinnamon , onion, garlic, black pepper, thyme, bay leaf, lavander, hyssop
Fluids	Hot tea made from oregano, mint, chamomile, milk, fenugreek, cinnamon, hibiscus tea

Table 10-1

Almond
Asparagus
Beef
Black pepper
Carrot
Cheese
Corn
Cucumber
Duck
Egg plant
Fig
Garlic
Ginger, dried
Grapes
Honey
Lettuce
Lotus root
Olive
Onion
Peanut
Pear
Radish
Radish seed
Rice
Salt
Loquat
Milk
Mushroom, butt
Mustard greens
Spinach
Swiss chard
Tangerine
Tofu
Walnut
Water chestnut
Watercress
Watermelon

Table 10-2

FIVE FLAVORS THAT AFFECT THE VITAL ORGANS

Organs	Flavors	Effects of Flavors
Liv/GB	Sour	Astringent
Ht/SI	Bitter	Strengthening
Sp/St	Sweet	Satisfying
Lu/LI	Pungent	Dispersing
Kid/UB	Salt	Softening
PC/TW	Bland	Regulating

Table 10-3

tion of your daily foods from the given lists that strengthen the lungs and respiratory system. make sure you are not allergic to them. Please treat them before you use.

EXERCISE

A certain amount of exercise is necessary to help improve circulation in order to distribute the nutrients to different parts of the body. Improved circulation will also help eliminate toxins. Lack of fluids and exercise can encourage the toxins to get trapped in the tissues, giving rise to various toxic syndromes.

In the beginning of treatment, if the patient is unable to exercise due to weakness, general body massages should be given. When the person is able to walk, regular walking should be encouraged. This can gradually be increased to brisk walking for ten minutes once or twice a day.

If the patient is able to do any other type of exercise (like aerobics, running, jogging, swimming, etc.) it should be encouraged.

Yoga exercises are gentle, and can be practiced by anybody, weak or strong. There are specific exercises and *Asanas,* that can be practiced to strengthen the lungs. Very weak patients should begin with one or two Yoga exercises until they are strong enough to add more into their schedule. Exercise is a good way to expel toxins from specific organs, to reduce stress, and to facilitate overall calmness. Yoga shouldn't be practiced without proper knowledge or guidance. People with reactions to aerobics or other type of exercises should consider learning Yoga. It is taught in schools and universities. There are many Yoga centers around the country. It would benefit you to go to one near you and learn the exercises properly from a reputable teacher.

Some type of exercise should be done regularly in order to promote healing and maintaining cardiovascular health. Overexertion or overdoing should be prevented by all means. Consistency and regularity will produce satisfactory results.

Nambudripad's Testing Techniques gave me the best tool to evaluate my patients with asthma, and NAET taught me the greatest healing technique to eliminate the problems, almost instantly and painlessly. NAET has truly revolutionized the practice of medicine! I applaud Dr. Devi for developing this unique technique and sharing it with the world. I have no doubt — this is going to be the "Medicine of the Future."

Robert Prince, M.D.
North Carolina

NAET has changed my life and practice. NAET is a profound and fascinating technique of correcting allergies, which is the underlying cause of most asthma and respiratory disorders.

NAET Sp: Sue Anderson, D.C.
Ann Arbor, MI
(734) 973-9692

Glossary

Acetaldehyde: An aldehyde found in cigarette smoke, vehicle exhaust, and smog. It is a metabolic product of Candida albicans and is synthesized from alcohol in the liver.

Acetylcholine: A chemical that transmits nerve impulses between cells. A neurotransmitter manufactured in the brain, used for memory and control of sensory input and muscular output signals.

Acid: Any compound capable of releasing a hydrogen ion; it will have a pH of less than 7.

Acute: Extremely sharp or severe, as in pain. Can also refer to an illness or reaction that is sudden and intense.

Acupuncture: An alternative medical treatment involving the insertion of special needles to treat illness and relieve pain.

Adaptation: Ability of an organism to integrate new elements into its environment.

Addiction: A dependent state characterized by craving for a particular substance if that substance is withdrawn.

Additive: A substance added in small amounts to foods to alter the food in some way.

Adrenaline: Trademark for preparations of epinephrine, which is a hormone secreted by the adrenal gland. It is used sublingually and by injection to stop allergic reactions.

Airways: The network of passageways that transport air in and out of the lungs during breathing.

Alveoli: Tiny air sacs deep inside the lungs where oxygen and carbon-di-oxide are exchanged during breathing.

Aldehyde: A class of organic compounds obtained by oxidation of alcohol. Formaldehyde and acetaldehyde are members of this class of compounds.

Alkaline: Basic, or any substance that accepts a hydrogen ion; its pH will be greater than 7.

Allergenic: Causing or producing an allergic reaction.

Allergen: Any organic or inorganic substance from one's surroundings or from within the body itself that causes an allergic response in an individual is called an allergen. An allergen can cause an IgE antibody mediated or non-IgE mediated response in a person. Some of the commonly known allergens are: pollens, molds, animal dander, food and drinks, chemicals of a different kind like the ones found in food, water, air, fabrics, cleaning agents, environmental materials, detergent, make-up products etc., body secretions, bacteria, virus, synthetic materials, fumes, and air pollution. Emotional unpleasant thoughts like anger, frustration, etc., can also become allergens and cause allergic reactions in people.

Allergic reaction: Adverse, varied symptoms, unique to each person, resulting from the body's response to exposure to allergens.

Allergic shiners: Dark circles under the eyes, usually indicative of allergies.

Allergy: Attacks by the immune system on harmless or even useful things entering the body touched by the skin, or breathed, etc. Abnormal responses to substances usually well tolerated by most people.

Amino acid: An organic acid that contains an amino (ammonia-like NH3) chemical group; the building blocks that make up all proteins.

Anaphylactic shock: Also known as anaphylaxis. Usually it happens suddenly when exposed to a highly allergic item; but sometimes, it can also happen as a cumulative reaction. (The first two doses of penicillin may not trigger a severe reaction, but the third or fourth one could produce an anaphylaxis in some people). An anaphylaxis (a life-threatening allergic reaction) is characterized by: an immediate allergic reaction that can cause difficulty in breathing, lightheadedness, fainting, sensation of chills, internal cold, severe heart palpitation or irregular heart beat, pallor, eyes rolling, poor mental clarity, tremors, internal shaking, extreme fear, angio-neurotic edema, throat swelling, drop in blood pressure, nausea, vomiting, diarrhea, swelling anywhere in the body, redness and hives, fever, delirium, unresponsiveness, or sometimes even death.

Antibody: A protein molecule produced in the body by lymphocytes in response to a perceived harmful foreign or abnormal substance (another protein) as a defense mechanism to protect the body.

Antigen: Any substance recognized by the immune system that causes the body to produce antibodies; also refers to a concentrated solution of an allergen.

Antihistamine: A chemical that blocks the reaction of histamine that is released by the mast cells and basophils during an allergic reaction. Any substance that slows oxidation, prevents damage from free radicals and results in oxygen sparing.

Assimilate: To incorporate into a system of the body; to transform nutrients into living tissue.

Autoimmune: A condition resulting when the body makes antibodies against its own tissues or fluid. The immune system attacks the body it inhabits, which causes damage or alteration of cell function.

Basophils: A type of white blood cell that mediates inflammatory reactions. They are functionally similar to mast cells and are found in mucous membranes, skin, and bronchial tubes.

B-cell: A white blood cell. It produces antibodies as directed by the T-cells.

Binder: A substance added to tablets to help hold them together.

Blood brain barrier: A cellular barrier that prevents certain chemicals from passing from the blood to the brain.

Bronchioloes: The smallest airways in the pulmonary system.

Bronchitis: Inflammation of the trachea and bronchi.

Bronchoconstriction: Tightening of the airways in the lungs.

Bronchodilators: Drugs that widen constricted airways.

Bronchospasm: A muscle contraction that lessens airflow in the lungs.

Buffer: A substance that minimizes changes in pH (acidity or alkalinity).

Candida albicans: A genus of yeast-like fungi normally found in the body. It can multiply and often cause severe infections, allergic reactions or toxicity.

Candidiasis: An overgrowth of Candida organisms, which are part of the normal flora of the mouth, skin, intestines and vagina.

Carbohydrate, complex: A molecule of sugar linked together, found in whole grains, vegetables, and fruits. This metabolizes into glucose slower than refined carbohydrate.

Carbohydrate, refined: A molecule of sugar that metabolizes quickly into glucose, e.g., white flour, white sugar, and white rice.

Cardiac Asthma: Breathing problems caused by fluid buildup in the lungs as a result of congestive heart failure.

Catalyst: A chemical that speeds up a chemical reaction without being consumed or permanently affected in the process.

Cerebral allergy: Mental dysfunction caused by sensitivity to foods, chemicals, environmental substances, or other substances like work materials etc.

Chemical Challenge: A test in which a suspected or known asthma trigger is inhaled and then a pulmonary function test is given to measure the degree of sensitivity present.

Congestive heart failure: A condition that occurs when the heart cannot pump enough blood to the lungs and the rest of the body, causing excess fluid to accumulate in the tissue.

Chronic: Of long duration.

Chronic fatigue syndrome: A syndrome of multiple symptoms most commonly associated with fatigue and reduced energy or no energy.

Crohn's disease: An intestinal disorder associated with irritable bowel syndrome, inflammation of the bowels and colitis.

Cumulative reaction: A type of reaction caused by an accumulation of allergens in the body.

Cyclic allergy: A type of allergy which, with abstinence and/or non-exposure, will disappear and will not reappear unless there is over-exposure to the substance.

Cystic fibrosis: A genetic disease that causes excess mucus production in the respiratory tract, leading to persistent infection of the lungs.

Cytokine: A chemical produced by the T-cells during an infection as our immune system's second line of defense. Examples of cytokines are interleukin 2 and gamma interferon.

Desensitization: The process of building up body tolerance to allergens by the use of extracts of the allergenic substance.

Detoxification: A variety of methods used to reduce toxic materials accumulated in body tissues.

Digestive tract: Includes the salivary glands, mouth, esophagus, stomach, small intestine, portions of the liver, pancreas, and large intestine.

Disorder: A disturbance of regular or normal functions.

Dust: Dust particles from various sources irritate sensitive individuals, causing different respiratory problems like asthma, bronchitis, hay fever-like symptoms, sinusitis, and cough.

Dust mites: Microscopic insects that live in dusty areas, pillows, blankets, bedding, carpets, upholstered furniture, drapes, corners of the houses where people neglect to clean regularly.

Eczema: An inflammatory process of the skin resulting from skin allergies causing dry, itchy, crusty, scaly, weepy, blisters or eruptions on the skin. Skin rash frequently caused by allergy.

Edema: Excess fluid accumulation in tissue spaces. It could be localized or generalized.

Electromagnetic: Refers to emissions and interactions of both electric and magnetic components. Magnetism arising from electric charge in motion. This has a definite amount of energy.

Elimination diet: A diet in which common allergenic foods and those suspected of causing allergic symptoms have been temporarily eliminated.

Emphysema: A disease of the alveoli that results in shortness of breath.

Endocrine: Refers to ductless glands that manufacture and secrete hormones into the blood stream or extracellular fluids.

Endocrine system: Thyroid, parathyroid, pituitary, hypothalamus, adrenal glands, pineal gland, gonads, the intestinal tract, kidneys, liver, and placenta.

Endogenous: Originating from or due to internal causes.

Endorphins: A natural substance produced in the brain that influences mood and perception of pain.

Environment: A total of circumstances and/or surroundings in which an organism exists. May be a combination of internal or external influences that can affect an individual.

Environmental illness: A complex set of symptoms caused by adverse reactions of the body to external and internal environments.

Enzyme: A substance, usually protein in nature and formed in living cells, which starts or stops biochemical reactions.

Eosinophil: A type of white blood cell that increases in number during an allergic reaction. Eosinophil levels may be high in some cases of allergy or parasitic infestation.

Epinephrine: A hormone produced by the adrenal gland.

Erythrocyte: Red blood cell.

Exercise challenge: A test involving physical exertion followed by a pulmonary function test to determine the presence of exercise induced asthma.

Exercise induced asthma: Breathing problem caused by exercise.

Exocrine: Refers to substance released through ducts that lead to a body compartment or surface.

Exogenous: Originating from or due to external causes.

Extracellular: Situated outside a cell or cells.

Extract: Treatment dilution of an antigen used in immunotherapy, such as food, chemical, or pollen extract.

Extrinsic asthma: Asthma caused by allergens in the environments.

Formaldehyde: A gas that irritates the airways; it is given off by such things as building materials, home furnishings, permanent-press clothing, cigarettes, liquid paper, carpets, name tags on fabrics, etc.

Fibromyalgia: An immune complex disorder causing general body aches, muscle aches, and general fatigue.

Fight or flight: The activation of the sympathetic branch of the autonomic nervous system, preparing the body to meet a threat or challenge.

Food addiction: A person becomes dependent on a particular allergenic food and must keep eating it regularly in order to prevent withdrawal symptoms.

Food grouping: A grouping of foods according to their botanical or biological characteristics.

Free radical: A substance with unpaired electrons, which is attracted to cell membranes and enzymes where it binds and causes damage.

Gene: The basic unit of heredity; each gene helps determine various inherited characteristics.

Gastrointestinal: Relating both to stomach and intestines.

Hay fever: Allergic reaction to airborne ragweed, and other pollens; symptoms include runny nose, sneezing, and itchy, watery eyes.

Heparin: A substance released during allergic reaction. Heparin has antiinflammatory action in the body.

Histamine: A body substance released by mast cells and basophils during allergic reactions, which precipitates allergic symptoms.

Holistic: Refers to the idea that health and wellness depend on a balance between physical (structural) aspects, physiological (chemical, nutritional, functional) aspects, emotional and spiritual aspects of a person.

Homeopathic: Refers to giving minute amounts of remedies that in massive doses would produce effects similar to the condition being treated.

Homeostasis: A state of perfect balance in the organism also called as Yin-Yang balance. The balance of functions and chemical composition within an organism that results from the actions of regulatory systems.

Hormone: A chemical substance that is produced in the body, secreted into body fluids, and is transported to other organs, where it produces a specific effect on metabolism.

Hydrocarbon: A chemical compound that contains only hydrogen and carbon.

Hypersensitivity: An acquired reactivity to an antigen that can result in bodily damage upon subsequent exposure to that particular antigen.

Hyperthyroidism: A condition resulting from over-function of the thyroid gland.

Hypoallergenic: Refers to products formulated to contain the minimum possible allergens: some people with few allergies can tolerate them well. Severely allergic people can still react to these items.

Hypothyroidism: A condition resulting from under-function of the thyroid gland.

IgA: Immunoglobulin A, an antibody found in secretions associated with mucous membranes.

IgD: Immunoglobulin D, an antibody found on the surface of B-cells.

IgE: Immunoglobulin E, an antibody responsible for immediate hypersensitivity and skin reactions.

IgG: Immunoglobulin G, also known as gammaglobulin, the major antibody in the blood that protects against bacteria and viruses.

IgM: Immunoglobulin M, the first antibody to appear during an immune response.

Immune system: The body's defense system, composed of specialized cells, organs, and body fluids that protects body from invaders and infections. . It has the ability to locate, neutralize, metabolize and eliminate unwanted or foreign substances.

Immunocompromised: A person whose immune system has been damaged or stressed and is not functioning properly.

Immunoglobulins: Any of five different antibodies that blocks the effects of antigens in the body.

Immunity: Inherited, acquired, or induced state of being, able to resist a particular antigen by producing antibodies to counteract it. A unique mechanism of the organism to protect and maintain its body against adversity of its surroundings.

Inflammation: The reaction of tissues to injury from trauma, infection, or irritating substances. Affected tissue can be hot, reddened, swollen, and tender.

Inhaler: A medication delivery device that allows medicine to be breathed directly into the lungs.

Inhalant: Any airborne substance small enough to be inhaled into the lungs; eg., pollen, dust, mold, animal danders, perfume, smoke, and smell from chemical compounds.

Intolerance: Inability of an organism to utilize a substance.

Intracellular: Situated within a cell or cells.

Intradermal: Method of testing in which a measured amount of antigen is injected between the top layers of the skin.

Intrinsic asthma: Asthma caused by another disease or condition.

Ion: An atom that has lost or gained an electron and thus carries an electric charge.

Kinesiology: Science of movement of the muscle.

Latent: Concealed or inactive.

Leukocytes: White blood cells.

Leukotrienes: A group of chemicals released from mast cells that cause harmful inflammation of the bronchi in asthma.

Lipids: Fats and oils that are insoluble in water. Oils are liquids in room temperature and fats are solid.

Lymph: A clear, watery, alkaline body fluid found in the lymph vessels and tissue spaces. Contains mostly white blood cells.

Lymphocyte: A type of white blood cell, usually classified as T-or B-cells.

Macrophage: A white blood cell that kills and ingests microorganisms and other body cells.

Masking: Suppression of symptoms due to frequent exposure to a substance to which a person is sensitive.

Mast cells: Large cells containing histamine, found in mucous membranes and skin cells. The histamine in these cells are released during certain allergic reactions.

Mediated: Serving as the vehicle to bring about a phenomenon. For example, an IgE-mediated reaction is one in which IgE changes cause the symptoms and the reaction to proceed.

Membrane: A thin sheet or layer of pliable tissue that lines a cavity, connects two structures, selective barrier.

Metabolism: Complex chemical and electrical processes in living cells by which energy is produced and life is maintained. New material is assimilated for growth, repair, and replacement of tissues. Waste products are excreted.

Migraine: A condition marked by recurrent severe headaches, often on one side of the head, often accompanied by nausea, vomiting, and light aura. These headaches are frequently attributed to food allergy.

Mineral: An inorganic substance. The major minerals in the body are calcium, phosphorus, potassium, sulfur, sodium, chloride, and magnesium.

Monocyte: A type of white blood cell.

Mucous membranes: Moist tissues forming the lining of body cavities that have an external opening, such as the respiratory, digestive, and urinary tracts.

Mucous glands: Glands embedded in the bronchial lining that keep airways lubricated with mucus so that harmful substances can be easily eliminated from the lungs.

Muscle Response Testing: A testing technique based on kinesiology to test allergies by comparing the strength of a muscle or a group of muscles in the presence and absence of the allergen.

NAET: (Nambudripad's Allergy Elimination Techniques)**:** A technique to eliminate allergies permanently from the body towards the treated allergen. Developed by Dr. Devi S. Nambudripad in 1983 and practiced by over 7,500 medical practitioners worldwide. This technique is completely natural, non-invasive, and drug-free. It has been effectively used in treating all types of asthma and allergies and problems arising from allergies. It is taught by Dr. Nambudripad in Buena Park, California to currently licensed medical practitioners. If you are interested and want to learn more about NAET or attend a seminar, please visit the website**:** www.naet.com.

Nasal polyp: Small fleshy growths inside the nose that may develop as a result of continuous inflammation of the mucous membrane.

Nervous system: A network made up of nerve cells, the brain, and the spinal cord, which regulates and coordinates body activities.

Neurotransmitter: A molecule that transmits electrical and/or chemical messages from nerve cell (neuron) to nerve cell or from nerve cell to muscle, secretory, or organ cells.

Nutrients: Vitamins, minerals, amino acids, fatty acids, and sugar (glucose), which are the raw materials needed by the body to provide energy, effect repairs, and maintain functions.

Occupational asthma: Asthma caused by exposure to allergen in the workplace.

Organic foods: Foods grown in soil free of chemical fertilizers, and without pesticides, fungicides and herbicides.

Outgassing: The releasing of volatile chemicals that evaporate slowly and constantly from seemingly stable materials such as plastics, synthetic fibers, or building materials.

Overload: The overpowering of the immune system due to massive concurrent exposure or to low level continuous exposure caused by many stresses, including allergens.

Parasite: An organism that depends on another organism (host) for food and shelter, contributing nothing to the survival of the host.

Parasympathetic nervous system: The part of the nervous system that tightens the bronchial tubes and decreases blood pressure and heart rates.

Pathogenic: Capable of causing disease.

Pathology: The scientific study of disease; its cause, processes, structural or functional changes, developments and consequences.

Pathway: The metabolic route used by body systems to facilitate biochemical functions.

Peak flow meter: An inexpensive, valuable tool used in measuring the speed of the air forced out of the lungs and helps to monitor breathing disorders like asthma.

Petrochemical: A chemical derived from petroleum or natural gas.

pH: A scale from 1 to 14 used to measure acidity and alkalinity of solutions. A pH of 1-6 is acidic; a pH of 7 is neutral; a pH of 8-14 is alkaline or basic.

Phenolics: (also known as terpenes). They are seen naturally in plants to give color and fragrance to the leaves, bark, flowers, fruits and saps. They are derivatives of benzene that are made synthetically, also to give flavor and color to foods and to help preserve them.

Postnasal drip: The leakage of nasal fluids and mucus down into the back of the throat.

Precursor: Anything that proceeds another thing or event, such as physiologically inactive substance that is converted into an active substance that is converted into an active enzyme, vitamin, or hormone.

Pulmonary disease: Diseases and conditions that affect the lungs, such as asthma, emphysema, and chronic bronchitis.

Prostaglandin: A group of unsaturated, modified fatty acids with regulatory functions.

Radiation: The process of emission, transmission, and absorption of any type of waves or particles of energy, such as light, radio, ultraviolet or X-rays.

RAST (radioallergosorbent assay: A laboratory test used to identify allergy to specific substances by measuring immunoglobulins E, (IgE, a protein found in white blood cells) levels in the blood.

Receptor: Special protein structures on cells where hormones, neuro-transmitters, and enzymes attach to the cell surface.

Respiratory system: The system that begins with the nostrils and extends through the nose to the back of the throat and into the larynx and lungs.

Rhinitis: Allergic inflammation of the mucous membrane that lines the nose.

Rotation diet: A diet in which a particular food and other foods in the same "family" are eaten only once every four to seven days.

Sensitivity: An adaptive state in which a person develops a group of adverse symptoms to the environment, either internal or external. Generally refers to non-IgE reactions.

Serotonin: A constituent of blood platelets and other organs that is released during allergic reactions. It also functions as a neurotransmitter in the body.

Sick building syndrome: (Also known as building materials related illness). This term is used when one or more occupants of a building develops similar symptoms related to some indoor pollutants. Many of these symptoms involve reactions to carpets, formaldehyde, pressed woods, paints, fiber glass, tile work, chemical cleansers, leaking gas from plastic and other synthetic materials.

Spirometer: An instrument used to measure the amount and speed of inhaled and exhaled from the lungs.

Spirometry: Tests of lung air capacity and pulmonary function performed with spirometer.

Status asthmaticus: A life-threatening, prolonged asthma attack.

Steroid: A substance of naturally occurring lipid molecules such as hormones, bile acids, precursors for vitamins, and certain natural drugs; in pharmacology, a synthetic compound used to suppress the action of the immune system.

Stress: Anything that places undue strain upon normal body functions. Stress may be internal in origin (disease, malnutrition, allergic reaction), or external (environmental factors).

Stridor: Noisy breathing, often caused by obstruction or inflammation of the larynx.

Sublingual: Under the tongue, method of testing or treatment in which a measured amount of an antigen or extract is administered under the tongue, behind the teeth. Absorption of the substance is rapid in this way.

Sulfites: A group of preservatives added to foods and medications that can trigger allergic asthma in some people.

Supplement: Nutrient material taken in addition to food in order to satisfy extra demands, effect repair, and prevent degeneration of body systems.

Susceptibility: An alternative term used to describe sensitivity.

Sympathetic nervous system: The part of the nervous system that raises blood pressure and heart rates and widens the bronchial tubes.

Symptoms: A recognizable change in a person's physical or mental state, that is different from normal function, sensation, or appearance and may indicate a disorder or disease.

Syndrome: A group of symptoms or signs that, occurring together, produce a pattern typical of a particular disorder.

Synthesis: Combining of separate elements and substances to make a new, coherent whole.

Synthetic: Made in a laboratory; not normally produced in nature, or may be a copy of a substance made in nature.

Systemic: Affecting the entire body.

Target organ: The particular organ or system in an individual that will be affected most often by allergic reactions to varying substances.

Tetrazine: (FD & C yellow dye # %): Food coloring known to cause an allergic asthma reaction in some people.

T-cell: A white blood cell that instructs B-cells to produce antibodies in an allergic reaction, or immune reaction.

Tolerance: The capacity of the body to withstand repeated exposure without symptoms.

Tolerance threshold: The maximum amount of allergens, stress, and exposures that an individual can tolerate without having symptoms.

Toxicity: A poisonous, irritating, or injurious effect resulting when a person ingests or produces a substance in excess of his or her tolerance threshold.

Toxin: Poisonous, irritating, or injurious substance.

Triggers: Irritants to the lungs that cause symptoms of asthma.

Resources

NAET Main Office
6714 Beach Blvd.
Buena Park, California 90621
http://www.naet.com
NAET website for all information regarding NAET
E. mail: naet@earthlink.net
(714) 523-0800; (714) 523-8900

Nambudripad Allergy
Research Foundation (NARF)
6714 Beach Blvd.
Buena Park, CA 90621
(714) 523-0800
E.mail: narfbp@hotmail.com
A Nonprofit foundation dedicated to NAET research

NAET Training Seminars
6714 Beach Blvd.
Buena Park, CA 90621
(714) 523-8900
http://www.naet.com
E. mail: naet@earthlink.net
NAET training information

General Health Organizations

These organizations provide free or reasonably priced printed materials, videotape, and educational programs on general aspects of asthma.

National Heart, Lung, and Blood Institute (NHLBI) Information Center
National Institute of Health (NIH)
P.O.Box 30105
Bethesda, Maryland 20824-0105
Phone: (301) 251-1222
Web Site: http://www.nhlbi.nih.gov/nhlbi/nhlbi.html

Gopher Site:
gopher://fido.nhlbi.nih.gov:70/11/nhlbi
Excellent national research resource and referral service; prepares helpful material, including booklets on starting an asthma support group and how to care for your child with asthma.

National Institute of Allergy and Infectious Disease
Office of Communications
Building No 31, Room 7A-50
31 Center Drive MSC
Bethesda, Maryland 20892-2520
Phone: (301) 496-5717
E.mail: ocpostoffice@flash.niaid.nih.gov
web site: http://.www.niaid.nih.gov
Researches causes, prevention, and treatment of allergies, provides pamphlets for people with asthma and their families. Write for information and catalog.

Asthma and Allergy Foundation of America (AAFA)
1125 15th Street NW, Suite 502
Washington D.C. 20005
Phone: (800) 7-ASTHMA or (202) 466-7643
Fax: (202) 466-8940
E.mail: info@aafa.org.
Web site: http://www.aafa.org
Produces bimonthly patient education newsletter filled with up-to-date asthma and allergy information; provides brochures and resource list of books and games that can be ordered at a discount to members.

American Lung Association (ALA)
1740 Broadway
New York, NY 10019-4374
Phone: (800) 565-5642
web site: http://www.lungusa.org

National Jewish Medical and Research Center
1400 Jackson Street
Denver, Colorado 80206-2762
Phone: (800) 222-5864 (Lung line is a hot line for callers to hear the most recent facts about asthma)
web site: http://www.njc.org

American College of Allergy, Asthma and Immunology (ACAAI)
85 West Algonquin Road, Suite 550
Arlington Heights, Illinois 60005
Phone: (847) 427-1200
Fax: (847) 427-1294
web site: http://allergy.mcg.edu

American Academy of Allergy, Asthma, and Immunology
611 East Wells Street
Milwaukee, Wisconsin 53202
Phone: (800) 822-2762
web site: http://www.aaaai.org

Allergy and Asthma Networks/Mothers of Asthmatics (AAN/MA)
3554 Chain Bridge Road, Suite 200
Fairfax, Virginia 22030-2709
Phone: (800) 878-4403
Web site: http://www.podi.com/health/aanma
Provides information, referrals, publication list of educational materials, sells peak flow meters, support organization.

American Academy of Medical Acupuncture
5820 Wilshire Blvd., Suite 500
Los Angeles, California 90036
Phone: (800) 521-2262
website: http://medicalacupuncture.org

American Chiropractic Association
1701 Clarendon Blvd.
Arlington, Virginia 22209
Phone: (703) 276-8800
Web Site: http://www.amerchiro.org

American Yoga Association
P O Box 19986
Sarasota, Fl 34276
Phone: (941) 953-5859

National Center for Homeopathy
801 North Fairfax Street, Suite 306
Alexandria, Virginia 22314
Phone; (703) 548-7790
Web Site; http://www.homeopathic.org

NAET Books and Products

Delta Publishing Company
6714 Beach Blvd.
Buena Park, CA 90621
(714) 523-0800
E-mail: naet@earthlink.net

Naeter Technology
6714 Beach Blvd.
Buena Park, CA90621
Fax: (714) 523-3068
Product available: Computer for Allergy Testing

Environmentally Safe Products

Quantum Wellness Center
Drs. Dave & Steven Popkin
1261 South Pine Island Rd.
Plantation, FL 33324
(954) 370-1900/ Fax: (954) 476-6281
E-mail: buddha327@aol.com

Cotton Gloves

Janice Corporation
198 US Highway 46
Budd Lake, NJ 07828-3001
(800) 526-4237

"Living Air" Air Filter

Martha Evans
(714) 541-3960
email: 928mevans@msn.com

Herbal Supplements
Kenshin Trading Corporation
1815 West 213th Street, Ste. 180
Torrance, CA 90501
(310) 212-3199

Phenolics
Frances Taylor/Dr. Jacqueline Krohn
Los Alamos Medical Center, Ste.136
3917 West Road
Los Alamos, NM 87544
(505) 662-9620

Enzyme Formulations, Inc
6421 Enterprise Lane
Madison, WI 53719
(800) 614-4400

Allergies Lifestyle & Health
205 Center Street, Ste. B.
Eatonville, WA 98328
(360) 832-0858
Health Products

Bio Meridian International
12411 S. 265 W. Ste. F
Draper, UT 84020
(801) 501-7517
Biomeridian Computer

Star Tech Health Services, LLC
1219 South 1840 West
Orem, Utah 84058
(888) 229-1114
Computerized Allergy Testing Services

Apex Energetics
1701 E. Edinger, Ste. A-4
Santa Ana, CA 92705
(714) 973-7733
Homeopathic Products

Thorne Research Inc.
P.O. Box 25
Denver, ID 83825
(208) 263-1337
Herbs and Vitamins

Oxy-Health Corporation
12007 Los Nietos Road, #9
Santa Fe Springs, CA 90670
(562) 906 8888
Health Products

Earth Calm
3805 Windermere Lane
Oroville, CA 95965
(530) 534 9982

Dreamous Corporation
12016 Wilshire Blvd. # 8
Los Angeles, CA 90025
(310) 442 8544

K & T Books
LAMC, Ste. 136
3917 West Road
Los Alamos, NM 87544
(505) 662 9620

Neuropathways EEG Imaging
427 North Canon Dr. # 209
Beverly Hills, CA 90210
(310) 276 9181

CHI/KHT
P.O. Box 5309
Hemet, CA 92544
(909) 766 1426
Health Products

Biochemical Laboratories
P.O.Box 157
Edgewood, NM 87015
(800) 545 6562

Green Healing Center
1700 Sansom St., Ste. 800
Philadelphia, PA 19103
215-751-9833
Herbs

Allergy Research Group
30806 Santana St
Hayward, CA 94544
800) 545 9960
Vitamins & Homeopathic products

QLT Corpn
3960 E. Palm Lane #9
Mesa, AZ 85215
(602) 617-1741

Life Source International
1007 Montana Ave. Ste. 125
Santa Monica, CA 90403
(310) 284 3565

Cache Creek Veterinary Service
15200 Country Road 96 B
Woodland Hills, CA 95695
(530) 666-7322

Life Gate Enterprises
25 Bridge St., Ste. # 7
Billerica, MA 01821
(978) 663-4400

Allergy Research Group
30806 Santana St.
Hayward, CA 94544
(800) 545-9960
Vitamins & Homeopathic products

Integrative Therapeutics, Inc.
9755 SW Commerce Cir., Ste. B2
Wilsonville, OR 97070
(503) 582-8386
Vitamin products

The Brain Garden
713 SE Everett Mall Way #D
Everett, WA 98208
(425) 290-5309
Organic and nutritious Food source

Garland Bookstore
176 Home Base Lane
Unityville, PA 17774

Energy Balance Resources
428 Mt. Davis Ave.
San Diego, CA 92117-3422
(866) 522-5262

BIBLIOGRAPHY

Abehsera, Michel, Ed., *Healing Ourselves,* 1973

Alan M. Weinstein, M.D., *Asthma,* Fawcett Crest Book, The Ballantine Publishing Group, 1987

Ali, Majid M.D., *The Canary and Chronic Fatigue,* Life Span Press, 1995

American Medical Association Committee on Rating of Mental and Physical Impairments, *Guides to the Evaluation of Permanent Impairment,* N.P., 1971

American Medical Association, *Essential guide to asthma,* pocket book, a division of Simon & Schuster Inc., 1230 Avenue of the Americas, New York, NY 10020, 1998

American Psychiatric Association, *Diagnostic and Statistical Manual of Mental Disorders,* 4th ed., 2000

American Thoracic Society, Standardization of Spirometry: 1994 update. *Am J Respir Crit Care Med* 1995; 152:1107-36.

Austin, Mary, *Acupuncture Therapy,* 1972

Batmanghelidj F., *ABC of Athma Allergies & Lupus*, Global health solutions, inc., falls Church, VA, 2000

Beasley R, Cushley M, Holgate ST. A self-management plan in the treatment of adult asthma. *Thorax* 1989;44:200-4.

Beeson, Paul B., M.D. and McDermott, Walsh, M.D., Eds., *Textbook of Medicine,* 12th edition, 1967

Bender, David, and Bruno Leone, *The Environment, Opposing Viewpoints,* Greenhaven Press, 1996

Blum, Jeanne Elizabeth, *Woman Heal Thyself,* Charles E. Tuttle Co., 1995

Brownstein, David, M.D., *The Miracle of Natural Hormones,* Medical Alternatives Press, 1998.

Brownstein, David, M.D., *The Miracle of Natural Hormones* 2nd edition. Medical 1996 Alternative Press, 1999

Brownstein, David, M.D., *Hormones and Chronic Disease,* Medical Alternative Press, 1999

Brownstein, David, MD., *Overcoming Arthritis*, Medical Alternative Press, 2001

Cecil Textbook of Medicine, 21st ed., 2000

Cerrat, Paul L., *Does Diet Affect the Immune System?,* RN, June 1990

Charlotte Shubert, *Burned by Flame Rretardants?* Science News, Vol. 160 , 2001

Chaitow, Leon, *The Acupuncture Treatment of Pain,* Thomsons Publishers, 1984

Charlton I, Charlton G, Broomfield J, Mullee MA. Evaluation of peak flow and symptoms only self-management plans for control of asthma in general practice. *BMJ*1990;301:1355-g

Collins, Douglas, R., MD., *Illustrated Diagnosis of Systematic Diseases,* 1972

Cousins, Norman, *Head First, The Biology of Hope and the Healing Power of the Human Spirit,* Penguin Books, 1990

Daniels, Lucille, M.A, and Catherine Wothingham, Ph.D., *Muscle Testing Techniques of Manual Examination,* 3rd ed., 1972

Davis, Rowland H., and Weller, Stephen G., *The Gist of Genetics,* Jones and Bartlett Publishers, 1996

East Asian Medical Studies Society, *Fundamentals of Chinese Medicine,* Paraadigm Publications, 1985

Elliot, Frank, A., F.R.C.P., *Clinical Laboratory*, 1959

Enright PL, Lebowitz, MD, Cockroft DW. Physiologic measures: pulmonary function tests. *Asthma outcome. Am J. Respir Crit Care Med* 1994; 149:59-18

Fazir, Claude A., MD., *Parents Guide to Allergy in Children,* Doubleday & Co., 1973

Fratkin, Jake, *Chinese Herbal Patent Formulas,* Institute of Traditional Medicine, 1986

Fujihara, Ken and Hays, Nancy, *Common Health Complaints,* Oriental Healing Arts Institute, 1982

Fulton, Shaton, *The Allergy Self Help Book,* Rodale Books, 1983

Gabriel, Ingrid, *Herb Identifier and Handbook,* Sterling Publishing Co., 1980

Gach, Michael Reed, *Acuppressure's Potent Points,* Bantam Books, 1990

Goldberg, Burton and Eds. of Alternative Medicine Digest, *Chronic Fatigue and Fibromyalgia & Environmental Illness*, Future Medicine Publishing, 1998

Goldberg, Burton and Eds. of Alternative Medicine Digest, *Definitive Guide to Headaches,* Future Medicine Publishing, 1997

Goodheart, George, J., *Applied Kinesiology,* N.P., 1964

---. *Applied Kinesiology*, 1970 Research Manual, 8th ed. N.P., 1971

---. *Applied Kinesiology*, 1973 Research Manual, 9th ed. N.P., 1973

---. *Applied Kinesiology*, 1974 Research Manual, N.P., 1974

---.*Applied Kinesiology*, Workshop Manual, N.P., 1972

Gray, Henry, F.R.S., *Anatomy of the Human Body,* 27th, 34th, and 38th eds., 1961

Graziano, Joseph, *Footsteps to Better Health,* N.P., 1973

Guyton, Arthur C., *Textbook of Medical Physiology,* 2nd ed., 1961

Haldeman, Scott, *Modern Developments in the Principles and Practice of Chiropractic,* Appleton-Century-Crofts, 1980

Hansel, Tim, *When I Relax I Feel Guilty,* Chariot Victor Publishing, 1979

Harris H., M.D., and Debra Fulghum Bruce, *The Fibromyalgia Handbook*, Holt and Co., 1996

Hepler, Opal, E., Ph.D., M.D., *Manual of Clinical Laboratory Methods,* 4th ed., 1962

Heuns, Him-Che., *Handbook of Chinese Herbs and Formulae,* Vol V., 1985

Hsu, Hong-Yen, Ph.D., *Chinese Herb Medicine and Therapy,* Oriental Healing Arts Institute, 1982

---. *Commonly Used Chinese Herb Formulas with Illustrations,* Oriental Healing Arts Institute, 1982

---. *Natural Healing With Chinese Herbs,* Oriental Healing Arts Institute, 1982

Janeway, Charles A., and Travers, Paul, and Walport, Mark, and Shlomchik, Mark, *Immunobiology*, Garland Publishing, 2001

Kandel, Schwartz, Jessell, *Principles of Neural Science,* McGraw Hill, 4th ed., 2000

Kennington & Church, *Food Values of Portions Commonly Used,* J.B. Lippincott Company, 1998

Kirschmann J.D. with Dunne, L.J., *Nutrition Almanac,* 2nd ed., McGraw Hill Book Co., 1984

Krohn, Jacqueline, M.D., and Taylor, Frances A., M.A. and Larson, Erla Mae, R.N., *Allergy Relief and Prevention*, 2nd. ed, Hartley & Marks, 1996

Krohn, Jacqueline, M.D., and Taylor, Frances A., M.A., *Natural Detoxification,* 2nd. ed, Hartley & Marks, 2000

Lawson-Wood, Denis, F.A.C.A. and Lawson-Wood, Joyce, *The Five Elements of Acupuncture and Chinese Massage,* 2nd ed., 1973

Lori Lite, *Welcome to NAET*, Lite Publishing, 2002

Lyght, Charles E., M.D., and John M. Trapnell, M.D., Eds., *The Merck Manual,* 11th ed., Merck Research Laboratories, 1966

MacKarness, Richard, *The Hazards of Hidden Allergies,* Mc Ilwain

Merkel, Edward K., and John, David T., and Krotoski, Wojciech A., Eds., *Medical Parasitology*, 8th. ed., W.B.Saunders Company, 1999

Milne, Robert, M.D., and More, Blake, and Goldberg, Burton, *An Alternative Medicine Definitive Guide to Headaches,* 1997

Mindell, Earl, *Vitamin Bible,* Warner Books, 1985

Moss, Louis, M.D., *Acupuncture and You,* 1964

Moyers, Bill, *Healing and the Mind,* Doubleday, 1976

Nambudripad, Devi, *Living Pain Free,* Delta Publishing Company, 1997

Nambudripad, Devi, *Say Good-bye to Illness, Spanish, 1st. ed.,* Delta Publishing Company, 1999

Nambudripad, Devi, *Say Good-bye to Illness, French, 1st. ed.,* Delta Publishing Company, 1999

Nambudripad, Devi, *Say Good-bye to Illness, English, 1st ed., 1993, 2nd. ed., 1999, 3rd. ed.,* 2002, Delta Publishing Company

Nambudripad, Devi, *Say Good-bye to ADD and ADHD,* Delta Publishing Company, 1999

Nambudripad, Devi, *Say Good-bye to Allergy-related Autism,* Delta Publishing Company, 1999

Nambudripad, Devi, *Say Good-bye to Children's Allergies,* Delta Publishing Company, 2000

Nambudripad, Devi, *Say Good-bye to Environmental Allergies,* Delta Publishing Company, 2003

Nambudripad, Devi, *Say Good-bye to Chemical Sensitivities,* Delta Publishing Company, 2003

Nambudripad, Devi, *Survivimg Biohazard Agents,* Delta Publishing Company, 2003

Nambudripad, Devi, *The NAET Guidebook,* 6th ed., Delta Publishing Company, 2001

Northrup, Christiane M.D., *Women's Bodies, Women's Wisdom,* Bantam Books, 1998

Palos, Stephan, *The Chinese Art of Healing,* 1972

Pearson, Durk, and Shaw, Sandy, *The Life Extension Companion,* Warner Books, 1984

Pert, Candace B., Ph.D., *Molecules of Emotion,* Scribner, 1997

Pitchford, Paul, *Healing with Whole Foods,* North Atlantic Books, 1993

Radetsky, Peter, *Allergic to the Twentieth Century,* Boston, Little, Brown and Co., 1997

Randolph, Theron, G., M.D., and Ralph W. Moss, Ph.D., *An Alternative Approach to Allergies,* Lippincott and Conwell, 1980

Rapp, Doris, *Allergy and Your Family,* Sterling Publishing Co., 1980

Rapp, Doris, *Is This Your Child?* Quill, William Morrow, 1991

Shanghai College of Traditional Chinese, *Acupuncture, a Comprehensive Text, 1999*

Shealy, C. Norman, M.D., Ph. D. and Caroline Myss, Ph. D., *The Creation of Health,* Stillpoint Publishing, 1993

Shima, Mike, *The Medical I Ching,* Blue Poppy Press, 1992

Shuttari MF. Asthma: *diagnosis and management. Am Fam Physian* 1995;52:2225-36

Sierra, Ralph, U., *Chiropractic Handbook of Applied Neurology,* Mexico, 1956

Somekh, Emile, M.D. *The Complete Guide To Children's Allergies,* Pinnacle Books, Inc., 1979

Smith, CW, *Electromagnetic Man: Health and Hazard in the Electrical Environment,* Martin's Press, 1989, 90, 97

Smith CW, Environmental Medicine: *Electromagnetic Aspects of Biological Cycles,* 1995:9(3):113-118

Smith CW., *Electrical Environmental Influences on the Autonomic Nervous System,* 11th. Intl. Symp. on *"Man and His Environ ment in Health and Disease"*, Dallas, Texas, February 25-28, 1993

Smith CW., *Electromagnetic Fields and the Endocrine System,* 10th. Intl. Symp. on *"Man and His Environment in Health and Disease"*, Dallas Texas, February 27- March 1, 1992

Smith CW., *Basic Bioelectricity: Bioelectricity and Environmental Medicine,* 15th. Intl. Symp., on *"Man and His Environment in Health and Disease",* Dallas, Texas, February 20-23, 1997. (Audio Tapes from: Professional Audio Recording, 2300 Foothill Blvd. #409, La Verne, CA

Spector SL, Nicklas RA, eds. *Practice parameters for the diagnosis and treatment of asthms. J Allergy Clin Immunol* 1995;96:729-31

Strunk RC. Asthma deaths in childhood: Identification of patients at risk and intervention. J Allergy Clin Immonol 1987;80:472-7

Sui, Choa Kok, *Pranic Healing*, Samuel Wiser, 1990

Stephanie Marohn, *The Natural Medicine Guide to Autism*, 1st Ed., Hampton Roads Publishing Company, 2002

Teitlebaum, Jacob, M.D., *From Fatigued to Fantastic,* 1st ed., 1996, 2nd. ed., 2001, Avery Penguin Putnam

Teitlebaum, Jacob, M.D., *Healing Through joy,* 1st edition, 2003, DEVA PRESS, Annapolis, MD,

Weiss, Jordan, M.D., *Psychoenergetics,* 2nd. ed., Oceanview Publishing, 1995

Zong, Linda, *Chinese Internal Medicine,* lectures at SAMRA University, Los Angeles, 1985

Case Histories from the Author's private practice, 1984-present

Index

D

E

F

K

L

M

N

O

P

R

S

BOOK ORDER FORM

Name of book	Price	Quantity	Total Price
Say Good-bye to Illness			
3rd. Edition (English)	$24.00	------------	--------------
Spanish Edition	$21.00	------------	--------------
French Edition	$24.00	------------	--------------
Say Good-bye to ADD &			
ADHD	$18.00	------------	--------------
Say Good-bye to Allery-Related Autism	$18.00	-----------	--------------
Say Good-bye to Children's Allergies	$18.00	------------	--------------
Say Good-bye to Your Allergies	$18.00	------------	--------------
Say Good-bye to Asthma	$18.00	------------	--------------
NAET Guide Book	$12.00	------------	--------------
Living Pain Free	$22.95	------------	--------------

Sales Tax	----------
S&H	----------
Total	----------

To order books, call:

(714) 523-8900 or (888) 890-0670
or send a check for the amount plus the applicable sales tax
and $5.00 for shipping and handling to:
Delta Publishing Company
6714 Beach Blvd.
Buena Park, CA 90621
Or vist the website: www.naet.com

BOOK ORDER FORM

Name of book	Price	Quantity	Total Price
Say Good-bye to Illness			
3rd. Edition (English)	$24.00	------------	--------------
Spanish Edition	$21.00	------------	--------------
French Edition	$24.00	------------	--------------
Say Good-bye to ADD & ADHD	$18.00	------------	--------------
Say Good-bye to Allery-Related Autism	$18.00	-----------	--------------
Say Good-bye to Children's Allergies	$18.00	------------	--------------
Say Good-bye to Your Allergies	$18.00	------------	--------------
Say Good-bye to Asthma	$18.00	------------	--------------
NAET Guide Book	$12.00	------------	--------------
Living Pain Free	$22.95	------------	--------------

Sales Tax	----------
S&H	----------
Total	----------

To order books, call:

(714) 523-8900 or (888) 890-0670
or send a check for the amount plus the applicable sales tax and $5.00 for shipping and handling to:

Delta Publishing Company
6714 Beach Blvd.
Buena Park, CA 90621
Or vist the website: www.naet.com